the insider's guide to
pregnancy

the insider's guide to
pregnancy
real mums tell it how it is

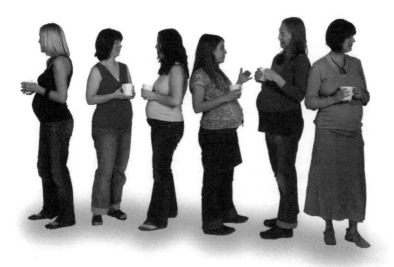

Editor: Stephen Giles

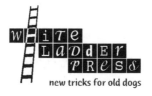

new tricks for old dogs

Published by White Ladder Press Ltd
Great Ambrook, Near Ipplepen, Devon TQ12 5UL
01803 813343
www.whiteladderpress.com

First published in Great Britain in 2007

10 9 8 7 6 5 4 3 2

ISBN 978 1 905410 11 8

British Library Cataloguing in Publication Data
A CIP record for this book can be obtained from the British Library.

Designed and typeset by Julie Martin Ltd
Cover design by Julie Martin Ltd
Cover photograph Jonathon Bosley

Printed and bound by TJ International Ltd, Padstow, Cornwall
Cover printed by St Austell Printing Company
Printed on totally chlorine-free paper

FSC (The Forest Stewardship Council) is an international
network to promote responsible management of the world's forests.

FSC
Mixed Sources
Product group from well-managed
forests and other controlled sources
Cert no. SGS-COC-2482
www.fsc.org
© 1996 Forest Stewardship Council

White Ladder books are distributed in the UK by Virgin Books

White Ladder Press
Great Ambrook, Near Ipplepen, Devon TQ12 5UL
01803 813343
www.whiteladderpress.com

ACKNOWLEDGMENTS

It is customary for this section to be a tribute to 'all those without whom it wouldn't have happened'. In this case that's the literal truth. Without the help, wit and wisdom of babyworld.co.uk members this book would not exist. All those who contributed deserve special thanks, including Leslie Schauerte, Amanda Bates, Steph Searle, Alix Alcott, Jessica Cather, Penny Goodyear, Marianne Monie, Kelly Tanner, Alexandria Matheson, Michelle Sudbury, Amanda Pearce, Marie Crutchley, Tracy Hill and Charlotte Johnston, everyone in the discussion forums and Sue and Steph. Thanks also to all at White Ladder and to midwife Sara Warren and Dr Ginny Cunliffe for their feedback in general and their specific focus on medical advice and recommendations. And special thanks to George for reminding me of anything I might have forgotten.

CONTENTS

babyworld.co.uk

babyworld.co.uk was born 10 years ago at the beginning of the internet revolution. We were bowled over by the intensity and speed at which **babyworld.co.uk** grew – we seemed to offer just the right potent mix of expert advice and personal experience our users craved. Our community and unique antenatal clubs rapidly became a honey pot for mums and dads seeking the holy grail of parenthood – to get through the parenting maze intact.

You are at the beginning of this maze with the worries and concerns that are the natural territory of pregnancy. Over the years, thousands of parents have offered each other fantastic advice, support and friendship on our site and it seemed selfish to keep it all to ourselves. Whilst there are so many sources of pregnancy information, the strongest of them, we hear time and again, is other parents' advice.

With our members' blessings, we decided to put their words of wisdom, from the antenatal clubs and pregnancy forums, into an insider's guide – a goldmine of advice from people you can trust.

babyworld.co.uk is a very big club, but it's surprisingly intimate in its knowledge of the trials and tribulations of becoming a parent. Only other parents can understand not only how much this job can take it out of you but also the rewards it brings. I can safely say that this message comes not just from me but from all the other parents who have contributed to this book: make the most of this time, whether it is your first or fifth foray into parenthood, and we hope that this book makes the journey just that bit more enjoyable.

Steph Neuman
Editorial Director of **babyworld.co.uk** and mum of two

FOREWORD

By Sue Allen-Mills
babyworld.co.uk antenatal clubs adviser

Pregnancy is a special and exciting time, but it can also be strange and bewildering. You may wonder if you're the only person experiencing what you're going through, whether it's normal, and what you might be able to do about it. Nobody understands this quite so well as someone else who's pregnant. And no one is better placed to empathise and offer practical suggestions than another pregnant woman. Pregnancy is also much more enjoyable if you're going through it with someone else, so that you can trade notes on aches and pains, share the high points, talk babytalk endlessly without the risk of boring the other person, and we all know what they say about a problem shared! Since 1999, thousands and thousands of women have had the opportunity of sharing their pregnancies on-line with others who are at the same stage of pregnancy as they are through *babyworld* antenatal clubs. Wherever they are, whatever time of day it is, if there's something they're worried about or would like advice or an opinion on, or if they've got some news they'd like to share, members can log on to their club and post a message, and others will soon respond with information, ideas, suggestions, or a listening ear.

This book draws on the extensive collective wisdom and experience of *babyworld* antenatal club members. It reflects the sorts of questions that commonly come up in the clubs and the wealth of answers that members have to give. It reveals what the experience of pregnancy is like for women themselves, and the sorts of strategies they adopt to see themselves through it. I hope it will show you that whatever it is that you're experiencing in your pregnancy, there are other women somewhere who are going through the same thing, who know what it's like, and who may have some tips for you. I hope too that it will give you a flavour of what it's like to be part of the *babyworld* community. Visit us at **www.babyworld.co.uk** to find out more.

INTRODUCTION

There is no such thing as an average pregnancy. And this is no average pregnancy book. The Insider's Guide to Pregnancy is put together from the hundreds of pregnancy experiences of the members of baby-world.co.uk – one of the UK's largest and most trusted websites on pregnancy and parenting issues.

Because it is drawn from the real life experiences of babyworld.co.uk members, this book provides a unique insight into the whole experience of pregnancy. It strips away the jargon and the patronising rhetoric of pregnancy textbooks to tell it how it is – from the positive pregnancy test all the way through to the delivery.

Divided into 100 bite-sized sections, with information on a massive range of pregnancy topics, this book contains thoughts, tips, advice and humour from a wide range of mums, from first-timers to fifth- or sixth-timers. Where more detailed medical advice is required, we have enlisted the help of our resident midwife.

In the spirit of the excellent babyworld.co.uk antenatal clubs, no subject is taboo and everyone's contribution is welcomed. Everyone has personal views on pregnancy and, just like any antenatal club, there's plenty of opinion here.

The contributions in this book aren't simply here to inform. They are included to entertain, to question and to spark debate. In reading them, I hope you find your own experiences are shaped by them and that they help your enjoyment and understanding of the remarkable, bewildering and unbeatable experience of pregnancy.

I hope you enjoy the journey – you're in great company.

Stephen Giles.

Important note:

While every effort has been made to check the factual accuracy of any medical opinion expressed in this work it is not designed to replace the advice of your midwife and/or GP. The advice contained in this book is, by its very nature, subjective, and neither White Ladder Press nor baby-world.co.uk assume any responsibility for any injuries, damages or losses suffered as a result of following this information.

"My period is late and I don't know whether I should do a home pregnancy test or go to the doctor – which is more accurate?"

THE PREGNANCY TEST

The most common way to test for pregnancy is with a home pregnancy test – these are extremely accurate and effective. They can be bought over the counter at chemists and supermarkets. If you prefer, a GP or Family Planning Clinic can do a pregnancy test, but the results may taker longer to be processed and, as they are less sensitive than home tests, may give a different result in the very early weeks.

You can take a pregnancy test just a few days after your missed period, though you may sometimes get a negative result when you're just one or two days late for your period and a strongly positive one when you're a week late. If you are pregnant, there's a sharp rise in the levels of the hormone that the test measures during this particular week

It is a good idea to take a test as soon as possible – when pregnancy is confirmed you can start to follow sensible dietary advice and take folic acid.

Babyworld.co.uk members on pregnancy tests:

▶ *Marli says:* 'My doctor told me that home pregnancy tests are eight times more sensitive than the hospital test so to take their results as gospel.'

▶ *Tula says:* 'I bought a load of pregnancy tests from a website called medisave.co.uk. You can buy ovulation kits online too and they cost a fraction of the branded ones in the shops. They are what is sold to medical clinics so they are top quality and you can choose the sensitivity ratings of them too.'

▶ *Peta says:* 'I found out last Thursday that I'm pregnant and find myself taking home tests every other day because the only symptom I have is sore boobs and that could be down to anything. But I keep smiling every time I see those two blue lines.'

▶ *Pip 180 says:* 'Most GPs send samples to hospital labs for testing (if they do tests at all, most now simply accept the results of a home test), and hospital tests are less sensitive, so you may not get a positive result until you're further on in your pregnancy.'

▶ *Ganeo says:* 'I did four tests because I didn't believe any of them and they were all huge dark blue crosses. Even then I took a picture and emailed it to all my friends and asked them to check!'

▶ *Marthasmum says:* 'A faint positive is a positive. I heard that if you've had a positive then get a negative result from a second test later in the day, it's because your urine tends to be more dilute as the day goes on. Tests work best on a sample of urine that's been in your bladder for at least four hours.'

See also:
Going to the doctor – page 8
Babyworld.co.uk link: **www.babyworld.co.uk/faq**

> **"Do I have to book an appointment with my GP at this early stage of pregnancy? If so, what should I expect?"**

GOING TO THE DOCTOR

With a first pregnancy, many women still expect a trip to the doctor will be the first 'confirmation' that they are pregnant. As we've seen, the home pregnancy test has made this initial appointment fairly redundant, certainly in terms of determining the existence of a pregnancy. In some areas of the UK a test will be done by the doctor or a urine sample will be taken, but these cases are in the minority as home tests are usually taken as authoritative proof.

You don't actually need to make an appointment to see the doctor at all. If you're not comfortable with the idea of seeing your doctor as the first 'official' recognition of your pregnancy, you can contact the midwife covering your area direct – get the number from your doctor's surgery or hospital antenatal clinic. It's unusual to be 'booked-in' by the midwife until 8-10 weeks, however, so if you feel the need to talk through any pregnancy concerns before this time, it's worth visiting the doctor who can give you information on dietary dos and don'ts as well as general information on your antenatal care.

If you have a history of problems in pregnancy, or if you have a specific medical condition that may affect your pregnancy, it is a good idea to get in touch with the doctor as soon as your pregnancy is confirmed. This will help you to get into the system at an early stage – giving you access to the specialist treatment you may need.

Babyworld.co.uk members on going to the doctor:

▶ *Mala says:* 'I visited the doctor and was just told to make an appointment to see the midwife at eight weeks and a scan at 12 weeks. The doctor didn't even congratulate me and I felt like I was just wasting her time. Definitely not going back to see the same one as she really deflated me.'

▶ *TeriP says:* 'Some GPs like to see women during pregnancy whereas others opt for midwife-only care unless there is a reason why a doctor needs to be seen. I haven't bothered with my GP, I've just booked to see the midwife.'

▶ *Anya3 says:* 'I saw my doctor at five weeks, and she filled in forms for my midwife care and to get me free NHS dental treatment and prescriptions.'

▶ *Rica says:* 'In my area you need to take a urine sample with you as the doctor confirms the pregnancy. At your follow-up appointment, when you get the results, you can discuss all your concerns.'

▶ *AimeeG says:* 'If you're aiming for a home birth my advice would be don't mention this to your GP – they can tend to be very negative about it, especially for first pregnancies. In actual fact a lot of GPs probably don't know enough about it to have a well formed opinion. Mention it at your first midwife appointment instead.'

▶ *Kyra37 says:* 'I saw my doctor just before I hit five weeks, and she was lovely – told me my due date, wished me luck and went through what I should be eating and not eating. She said to either call or come back if I had any questions or problems.'

▶ *GisellePG says:* 'With my first three pregnancies the GP accepted my word for being pregnant. With my fourth the GP did the test in his office with their own home testing kit, then with my fifth and sixth I've had to take in a urine specimen to be sent to the hospital for testing.'

See also:

The pregnancy test – page 6
Antenatal appointments – page 146
Babyworld.co.uk link: **www.babyworld.co.uk/faq**

"I feel different, but how do I know these symptoms are pregnancy related?"

BREAST SENSITIVITY AND OTHER EARLY SIGNS

For most women, the first hint that they might be pregnant is a missed period. But there are other early indications – if your breasts feel swollen or tender and you feel sick, an increased need to urinate and extreme tiredness, you can be fairly sure you are pregnant.

Of course, not all women experience all of these symptoms – and certainly not at the same stages. But generally some or all of these symptoms will affect most women to some degree over the first dozen weeks of pregnancy or so. Breast tenderness is usually noticeable from weeks three or four, sickness may also start in the first four weeks, but generally becomes more troublesome in the second and third month.

Breast tenderness often eases at around 12 weeks of pregnancy, nausea at around 14 weeks. This is quite normal. It doesn't mean that there is anything wrong with your hormones or your pregnancy. Your breasts will continue to grow throughout pregnancy, but most of the major changes to prepare your breast for breastfeeding will have occurred in the first couple of months. Nausea may return in waves at different stages of pregnancy – particularly in the later months.

Babyworld.co.uk members on early signs:

▶ *Gela says:* 'I got loads of symptoms from the first week I knew I was pregnant – sore boobs, sickness at four every morning, my waistline has disappeared, I have constipation and tiredness. Pregnancy is not for the faint-hearted!'

▶ *Jax says:* 'I've been told that feeling hot is a common early pregnancy symptom and that boob tenderness actually tends to be more pronounced in first pregnancies than in subsequent ones. As for sickness, this often doesn't start till around six weeks, though some women experience it earlier.'

▶ *Tula says:* 'I am feeling really tired at the moment and my nausea comes and goes. I keep getting headaches and feeling dizzy and I've only known I'm pregnant for a few days!'

▶ *LaraP says:* 'My symptoms are coming on nicely. I have a horrible taste in my mouth, really sore boobs, feeling very sick and so, so tired. I'm feeling good and pregnant in fact!'

▶ *Kentlass says:* 'The only symptoms I have at the moment are sore and heavy boobs (which have gone up one size already) and I am very tired. Over the last couple of nights I have felt a bit sick in the evening but that might be down to being so tired.'

▶ *MayaM says:* 'I have bigger boobs, they don't feel any different though. I've just started feeling nauseous especially before lunch and before my evening meal along with feeling hungry at the same time. I'm also bloated and my hips and legs ache when I do any physical activity.'

▶ *Suze says:* 'From as soon as I found out I was pregnant at about five weeks up until eight weeks I was physically shattered, and between 2-4pm every day I really couldn't function at all and needed to rest.'

See also:
Lack of symptoms – page 12
Fluctuating symptoms – page 14
Morning sickness and nausea – page 20
Swollen and sore breasts – page 32
Babyworld.co.uk link: **www.babyworld.co.uk/faq**

"The test was positive, but I don't 'feel' pregnant. When is it going to start?"

LACK OF SYMPTOMS

Midwife says: There are many factors that influence the range and intensity of symptoms that you experience in pregnancy. Anything from age to working environment via state of health, what you're eating, previous pregnancies, whether you smoke or not, and how your body reacts to pregnancy hormones can have an impact on how many symptoms you experience, when they arise, and how long they last.

The important thing to remember is that if you are feeling well and are not experiencing any danger signs – bleeding or severe cramping – then there is very probably nothing to worry about if you don't have any symptoms in the early weeks. 'Feeling' pregnant, which is an indefinable instinct that might be linked to the start of hormonal changes, is something that some women experience, but by no means all do.

Other symptoms vary too. While some women are hit by a tidal wave of symptoms, such as sickness, tiredness and aches and pains, right from the start, for others symptoms like sickness don't kick in till around six weeks, or even later. Sometimes sickness comes and goes, while a minority of women escape it entirely. There is no set pattern, and there's certainly nothing you can do to 'bring on' your symptoms. My advice is to enjoy the calm while it lasts.

Babyworld.co.uk members on lack of symptoms:

▶ *Pol02 says:* 'The extent to which women experience pregnancy symptoms is variable, and some women don't have any at all, so a lack of symptoms doesn't necessarily mean that there's anything wrong. This can be a worrying stage if you don't have any clear indications that you're pregnant, though if you've had no pain or bleeding, it would suggest that all's likely to be well with your baby.'

▶ *Marthasmum says:* 'I am pregnant with my third child, and once again I have no symptoms apart from slightly tender breasts when I first wake up. With my first two pregnancies I didn't have any symptoms in the early days, but I was sick as a dog for 10-15 days at 17 weeks when it's all meant to be over.'

▶ *TelZ says:* 'Not everyone has symptoms in the early weeks, and it's quite normal not to feel sick, not to have sore boobs, and not to have put any weight on at this stage – lots of women actually lose weight in early pregnancy.'

▶ *Brumb says:* 'I had no symptoms whatsoever with my son. I used to pray for morning sickness just to show things were going along OK.'

▶ *Peta says:* 'I didn't have sickness until six weeks, and I have friends who didn't get it at all – even one who didn't know she was pregnant until nine weeks as she had no symptoms! It doesn't mean anything bad, our bodies just react differently.'

See also:
Fluctuating symptoms – page 14
Babyworld.co.uk link: **www.babyworld.co.uk/faq**

"Last week I had everything – morning sickness, sore breasts and tiredness. This week I feel normal. Have I lost my baby, or is it normal for symptoms to stop?"

FLUCTUATING SYMPTOMS

The symptoms of pregnancy can be a cause of considerable stress and confusion in the early days and weeks of pregnancy. Many women find themselves analysing even the slightest change in mood or feeling in case it is an indication of something more sinister.

Fluctuating symptoms can be particularly worrying for women in the early stages. Many express concerns that the sudden absence of symptoms points to miscarriage or to an ectopic pregnancy. But if you aren't experiencing any danger signs – bleeding or sharp pains – then your fluctuating symptoms are unlikely to be a cause for concern.

Right now the experience of pregnancy can feel like a rollercoaster, with a whole range of new and uncomfortable sensations. But rest assured most women find their symptoms level out to a more manageable rate from the beginning of the second trimester.

Babyworld.co.uk members on fluctuating symptoms:

▶ *MegsT says:* 'It's not at all unusual for symptoms to fluctuate, especially in the first few weeks – some women won't have any symptoms at all at this stage. It's also quite normal to feel emotional, and for your mood to be all over the place.'

▶ *Ella3 says:* 'My symptoms started around six weeks, went away around seven, and started again at nine. I think I have learned that not all pregnancies are the same!'

▶ *Mia says:* 'When I miscarried, I actually stopped experiencing symptoms around eight weeks, even though I didn't miscarry until

13 weeks. If your symptoms disappear for weeks on end that can be a real worry.'

▶ *Kentlass says:* 'My symptoms come and go, I had no sore boobs first thing today, I kept on prodding them, desperately trying to find pain. Then about an hour later, it came back with a vengeance. We moan when we have symptoms but wish we had them when they disappear – all part of pregnancy I guess!'

▶ *Prio says:* 'Not feeling yourself is a good indication that everything's OK, in my book. I've been feeling 'odd' for a while. My sickness comes and goes – I haven't had severe morning sickness like some people I know, and I'm having twins, which is supposed to make it worse.'

▶ *MaisieK says:* 'My sickness often disappears for a couple of days at a time, then I worry, then it's back and I'm wishing it was gone. I'm going through a 'no sickness' phase at the moment, and so I'm panicking. I also feel my boobs are nowhere near as painful, but that does coincide with buying a soft cup bra without underwire.'

▶ *Spainbabe says:* 'I was really fed up with my disappearing and reappearing symptoms so I went to see my GP and said I wanted a scan so I could know what was going on. I thought she'd be as unsympathetic as my midwife but she said the most important thing was to reassure me. She offered to book me a scan and rang me at home within half an hour to say she'd persuaded them to start a few minutes early the next day so I could have one.'

See also:
Lack of symptoms – page 12
Fear of miscarriage – page 92
Miscarriage – page 94
Ectopic pregnancy – page 96
Babyworld.co.uk link: **www.babyworld.co.uk/faq**

> **"I've been getting cramps on and off over the last few weeks. Does this mean I'll miscarry?"**

PERIOD-LIKE CRAMPS

Midwife says: Cramps can be worrying, especially as they can be a sign of miscarriage, but not all cramps are associated with miscarrying. They are actually very common in the early weeks of pregnancy, and as long as they're mild and intermittent – not severe or persistent – they're unlikely to be a sign of anything being wrong.

There are a number of things that can cause cramping, and it's not always possible to be one hundred per cent sure of their cause in any one particular case. They may be 'stretching' pains as the uterus starts to grow, or be due to the uterus reacting to the presence of the embryo or to hormonal changes, or they may be associated with a urine infection or constipation, both of which are common in pregnancy.

Whatever the cause of these period-like cramps, remember that your body is experiencing huge changes in the first few weeks of pregnancy, and these changes may involve occasional mild discomfort. Please be reassured that this is a harmless part of the natural process. If you're experiencing severe cramping, however, this should be reported to your GP or midwife.

Babyworld.co.uk members on period-like cramps:

▶ *Han67 says:* 'I read that pain in the lower abdomen and pelvis can be from the corpus luteum in your ovary, which produces pregnancy hormones throughout the first ten weeks.'

▶ *Teri says:* 'I am getting quite annoying pains at the moment. They are mainly in the evening when I am really tired and they seem to have gone by the morning. I'm sure that it is normal and just my baby growing. The uterus expands a lot in the first trimester even though I can't see it yet.'

▶ *Peto says:* 'It's only when you have spotting and continued cramp that it could be something more serious. My best friend had bad cramps at the beginning of her pregnancy – and she is 26 weeks now.'

▶ *Mags01 says:* 'I had these sort of pains at a similar stage in my last pregnancy and rushed off to the doctor all worried. He explained that it's quite common to get pains in early pregnancy – if you get any bleeding however (fresh red blood or dark red blood, but not old brown stuff) you should see a doctor right away.'

Cramps in later pregnancy

● While period-like cramps are most common in the early weeks of pregnancy, they can occur at other stages of pregnancy too. They're generally not anything to worry about, but if they persist or are severe, it would be wise to let your midwife or GP know about them, as cramping can sometimes be a sign of a urine infection. And if they fall into a regular pattern, getting closer together and longer and stronger, contact your hospital, as you might be in labour.

● Some women experience cramps during orgasm in pregnancy. As long as there's not a severe pain, this is also perfectly normal. As the uterus is enlarged in pregnancy, the muscular contractions of the uterus during orgasm may affect other organs nearby. If you encounter sharp pains, or bleeding as a result of the cramps, consult your midwife or GP.

See also:
Thrush – page 30
Miscarriage – page 94
Babyworld.co.uk link: **www.babyworld.co.uk/faq**

> "I know I'm meant to be excited about my pregnancy, but I'm just too worried about what can go wrong to enjoy a single moment."

FEELING ANXIOUS

Lots of women feel this way, though few will be brave enough to admit to it – especially if they've been trying for a baby for a long time, or have been through the nightmare of a miscarriage in the past. Society expects a lot from mums-to-be, you're meant to be in a state of constant bliss, but that's simply not realistic.

Hormones play a part and you may feel less anxious as your new hormone levels settle down. But it is perfectly reasonable to feel anxious about a new phase in your life in which another person will depend on you in a way you have probably never experienced.

Pregnancy marks a change in your relationship with your partner, family and friends, as well as your career and body. Anxiety reflects the fact that you're treating these changes seriously. It is vital that you deal with any concerns you raise at this time – by speaking to friends, family or maybe someone at a bit of a distance, your GP, or other women in a similar situation on web discussion forums.

Babyworld.co.uk members on anxiety:

▶ *Loli says:* 'I don't think there are any magic solutions to feeling like this, as it's really all about what's going on in your mind, but you might find that it helps just to take things one day at a time, and to see each day as bringing you a day closer to your baby being born, and/or to try and focus on the 'what is's' rather than the 'what ifs'. The what is's are actually happening, whereas the what ifs may well not ever happen.'

▶ *Trem89 says:* 'Partly I'm worried about getting really huge, and pregnancy problems, partly about the pain of giving birth, but mostly about what on earth I am going to do with a baby – I am not even sure how to change a nappy.'

▶ *MSP says:* 'When I was feeling really anxious, my sickness became much worse and that could have been because of the way I was feeling emotionally. If there's any way you can do something to take your mind off things it might help.'

▶ *Megansmummy says:* 'I have been quite anxious as I've previously had a miscarriage, and my pregnancy symptoms have been extremely mild – sometimes non-existent. When I had an early scan, I was so scared, imagining the worst. There on the screen I saw tiny little bean with heart beating. I cried – I couldn't believe it. I am feeling much more positive and am ready to embrace and believe all will continue well.'

▶ *Tula says:* 'Worry is normal, especially if you've experienced loss or those around you have. And when you're part of internet groups and forums, you meet more pregnant people than you normally would, so you meet more that have lost babies. This makes it seem like it is more common than it is which increased my worry. Doesn't make it any easier that others worry just the same.'

You aren't alone

Most women find their mood lifting as the weeks go by, but a few find themselves sinking deeper into real depression. If you feel this is happening to you, speak with your midwife or doctor. 'Antenatal depression' is now a recognised condition – like postnatal depression – and safe treatment is available.

See also:

Mood swings – page 42
Your changing appearance – page 116
Babyworld.co.uk link: **www.babyworld.co.uk/faq**

> **"I've been feeling sick on and off for a few weeks – when will it stop and how can I ease it?"**

MORNING SICKNESS AND NAUSEA

If ever a pregnancy complaint needed investigating under the Trades Descriptions Act it's 'morning sickness'. It could just as easily be called 'all-day vomiting', 'afternoon queasiness' or 'evening heaves'. And for between 20 and 30 per cent of pregnant women it means absolutely nothing, as they avoid it all together. But everyone else will experience nausea on a sliding scale of severity from early days through to 10-14 weeks or beyond.

A sizeable minority of women experience sickness or nausea throughout pregnancy. For some it comes in waves, triggered by a particular activity – like getting out of bed or brushing teeth, for others it's a permanent fixture, mainly held at bay by sticking to the rule of eating little and often. Sickness in late pregnancy isn't so unusual, and this can be one of the early signs that your body is preparing for labour.

The cause of all this unease is unclear – certainly hormonal changes come into play, as do changes in blood pressure, digestive system and senses. The good news from all of this upheaval is that pregnancy nausea is linked to a reduced risk of miscarriage. But like all symptoms, extreme and prolonged cases of sickness, especially copious vomiting, will require medical attention.

Babyworld.co.uk members on morning sickness and nausea:

▶ *GabyK says:* 'Ginger is supposed to really help ease sickness but you may find that the bubbles in ginger ale/beer give you indigestion. Try ginger cordial – it is really good and you can make it up hot or cold. Without the bubbles it is great for morning sickness.'

▶ *Maya6 says:* 'With our daughter I had really bad sickness. I couldn't eat at all in the mornings, which would make me feel weak in the afternoons. The best thing to do is lie in bed for 10 minutes, eat a plain digestive biscuit and get up slowly.'

▶ *Hari says:* 'Green tea seems to work.'

▶ *Suki says:* 'I find a stash of sweets helps. When a wave of nausea hits or I know I'm about to go into a situation that may make me feel nauseous, eating something like that helps, partly, I think, as I munch them a lot so it's becoming a very familiar taste.'

▶ *Mum2B says:* 'Some women become ultra sensitive to smells, and there's no magic solution to this problem, though I have known women who've found that sniffing a cut lemon has helped.'

▶ *Krystal says:* 'I started taking ginger capsules for morning sickness and it brought near total relief.'

More tips to beat nausea

- Eat regular snacks rather than large meals – think 'little and often'.

- Stick to bland and dry foods (bread, crackers, fruit and vegetables). Avoid rich, fatty and spicy food.

- Homeopathic remedies, acupressure and acupuncture may all help to ease nausea. Consult a qualified practitioner for advice.

- Travel sickness wristbands can sometimes prove effective, though you should avoid over-the-counter travel sickness medicines without consulting your GP first.

See also:
Cravings – page 22
Toothcare and bleeding gums – page 50
Severe sickness and hyperemesis – page 72
Babyworld.co.uk link: **www.babyworld.co.uk/faq**

"I was absolutely desperate for a bacon sandwich this morning – but I hate bacon, always have!"

CRAVINGS

Hankering after bizarre combinations of food is supposedly one of the main signs of pregnancy, but the reality is that few women experience extreme cravings. As pregnancy affects your sense of taste and smell it is quite common to suddenly take against a favourite food or discover a passion for something new. But there seems to be no medical basis for the particular food chosen, indeed some experts suggest the choice has more to do with emotion – seeking comfort in a favourite childhood meal or 'reward' treat and developing an aversion to 'risk' foods like coffee and alcohol.

Sweet foods feature strongly on the list of must-haves, which is why it is essential to manage cravings as part of a balanced diet. Eating too much of any one food is likely to push out other food groups and may lead to health problems – though if your cravings are too strong to beat and your diet becomes imbalanced, it is worth consulting your GP or midwife for suitable vitamin supplements.

Babyworld.co.uk members on cravings:

▶ *EllieB says:* 'I can't get enough of chips and ice-cream (together) at the moment. Chips MUST be hot and salty, ice-cream MUST be vanilla and fairly soft!'

▶ *Fedor says:* 'I was in the supermarket one Saturday when it was pretty busy and had an urge to go over to the potatoes with all the dirt on them and lick them. My partner caught me in the nick of time and asked what I was doing – I said I was smelling them.'

▶ *Kayla says:* 'I love making biscuits, mixing all the ingredients and then cooking it and feeling like I am all domesticated. My husband suggested I try and get the same satisfaction from steaming vegetables but it isn't the same.'

The downside of cravings

- Craving banned foods – being desperate for it doesn't suddenly put it back on the menu. Remember the eating guidelines issued by your midwife – avoid shellfish, raw or undercooked meat, liver and liver products, fresh pate and ripened and blue cheeses. Cream cheeses and spreads are fine, because they are processed.

- Pica – this is the term given to cravings for non-food items – soil, coal, soap etc. No matter how strong your craving, you must divert yourself from it, possibly with a tasty treat. In its extreme form, pica can be masking an underlying physical or mental problem, so if you are struggling to resist, consult your GP or midwife.

- Allergy triggers – peanuts are a recurring theme in many women's craving stories. Experts advise women to avoid eating peanuts in pregnancy if there's any family history of nut allergies, asthma or eczema.

See also:
Smoking, drinking and drugs – page 118
Babyworld.co.uk link: **www.babyworld.co.uk/faq**

"I seem to be suffering discomfort after every meal – and even at other times. Am I eating the wrong things, and is there anything my doctor can give me?"

HEARTBURN AND INDIGESTION

Indigestion in general and heartburn in particular are extremely common in pregnancy. There's a two-pronged attack on your digestion, coming both from the detrimental effect of pregnancy hormones on the muscular opening at the top of your stomach and from pressure applied to the stomach by the expanding uterus.

Like its equally unappealing siblings constipation and flatulence, heartburn is kept under control with a good diet and regular exercise. Antacid is also available in liquid and tablet form for the effective treatment of heartburn, but you should consult your doctor first (it's also cheaper on prescription).

Heartburn can also be brought on by stress, by rushing your meals, or by doing too much straight after a meal. It might just sound like something you mother would say, but it really does make sense to 'let your dinner go down' by sitting for a while after each meal.

Babyworld.co.uk members on heartburn:

▶ *JazP says:* 'I have found that some foods help, if the heartburn is not too bad. Almonds, coconut and mango seem to be the best (I make myself a little fruit and nut mix snack in the afternoon – this seems to stave off the heartburn until after tea!). Logically, alkaline foods should help to counteract the acid that causes heartburn. I have read that almonds and coconuts are both quite alkaline.'

▶ *Peto says:* 'I get Gaviscon on prescription but if that doesn't work I eat a slice of dry bread which usually does the trick.'

▶ *Marthasmum says:* 'I did hear once that mint can help – I used to get heartburn all the time and drank mint cordial which did seem to help a bit.'

▶ *Luca says:* 'I'm guzzling milk like a crazy person, sometimes it helps a little. I've heard that a slice of fresh pineapple after a meal can help.'

▶ *Pip180 says:* 'Peppermint tea definitely works a treat. It is fantastic. If I have it too soon after eating then it messes everything up and I get heartburn again, but timed just right it really does help me. Apparently you should always eat something raw with your food to help aid digestion – this might be why the raw tomato seems to help me. I have just made sure that I have a little tomato salad on the side of dinner.'

▶ *Suse says:* 'I don't drink for at least half an hour after taking Gaviscon as the fluid seems to lie on top of the Gaviscon and makes me feel worse. Avoid tea, coffee and chocolate (and alcohol) as they relax the valve at the top of the stomach and make things worse.'

▶ *Suki says:* 'If other remedies aren't working try taking a couple of paracetamol as sometimes pain from muscular stretching and rib expansion can feel a bit like heartburn.'

See also:
Constipation – page 44
Flatulence – page 48
Smoking, drinking and drugs – page 118
Keeping fit and exercising – page 120
Babyworld.co.uk link: **www.babyworld.co.uk/faq**

"I've been suffering from regular headaches, but I'm not keen on taking painkillers. What can I do to ease them?"

HEADACHES

Headaches are common in pregnancy for a number of reasons. Firstly, the pesky pregnancy hormone progesterone may be responsible, as it can widen the blood vessels in the brain, leading to pounding headaches. There's nothing sinister at work here, and paracetamol (which is safe to use in pregnancy) should help to clear these up. Avoid using paracetamol too frequently, however, as a recent study has shown that pregnant women who took paracetamol 'on most days' were more likely to have a baby that wheezes.

Hormones are not the only source of headaches in pregnancy. Some women experience changes to their eyes which mean their contact lenses no longer fit properly or their glasses may not be suitable. In some cases, headaches may be linked to low blood sugar. If you're experiencing headaches in the long breaks between meals, try eating something starchy (bread, rice or pasta) in small, regular portions.

By far the most common source of headaches is stress. The pressure from tense shoulder and neck muscles puts more pressure on the scalp muscles and a headache is rarely far behind. The solution is not to get stressed of course, but that's easier said than done during pregnancy. But these headaches can be eased by closing your eyes, taking deep, calming breaths and massaging your temples. Lavender oil is a natural relaxant, but should only be used in the last three months of pregnancy.

Finally, a note of caution. Headaches may sometimes be related to high blood pressure and pre-eclampsia – especially from 20 weeks onwards. Though your BP should be checked regularly at antenatal appointments, if you are worried about headaches, you should contact your GP for a check-up.

Babyworld.co.uk members on headaches:

▶ *Maxi says:* 'I've tried using cooling gel packs. Also soaking your hands in warm water can help as well as it increases blood flow to the brain.'

▶ *Karla3 says:* 'Some headaches are triggered by fast dehydration so keeping fluids higher than normal may help.'

▶ *Lula says:* 'Rather than relying on paracetamol, I now try to drink more water and eat lots of small snacks throughout the day.'

▶ *Mum2B says:* 'I've been getting stinking headaches all through my pregnancy at the times when I would usually be due my period, so there is obviously something weird going on with hormones.'

▶ *FranM says:* 'I had lots of headaches when I cut out caffeine. They took about two weeks to go I think. I tried using half caffeine and half normal coffee for a while.'

▶ *Teri says:* 'The only thing I found has helped is a lavender heat cushion. You pop it in the microwave for a few minutes. Using lavender oil in a burner is good too.

▶ *Luca says:* 'I find that staying cool and using a nice cold gel eye mask that's been in the fridge helps.'

▶ *TrixB says:* 'I find that I get a headache around mid-morning. If I eat a banana it seems to adjust my blood sugars and I'm OK again.'

See also:
Getting ill – page 98
Pre-eclampsia – page 106
Keeping fit and exercising – page 120
Trying alternative remedies – page 136
Babyworld.co.uk link: **www.babyworld.co.uk/faq**

"I have had quite an increase in discharge – I'm panicking that there could be something wrong"

VAGINAL DISCHARGE

The first thing to stress is that increased vaginal discharge is common in pregnancy – it's rarely an indication of a problem with the baby. There are many factors contributing to the increase in discharge from the vagina in pregnancy. The blood supply increases, the cervix and vaginal walls soften, and in later stages, the baby's head pushes against the cervix in preparation for labour.

That doesn't make the idea of increased discharge any more cheering, or any less worrying when – as can happen – there is a sudden increase in discharge. This can sometimes happen after a period of heavy activity, such as walking or exercising. Normal discharge is clear, white or creamy in colour with a fairly runny consistency and no unpleasant odour. If the discharge thickens, becomes greenish or develops a foul smell, there may be an infection which will require medical attention. Most vaginal infections (like thrush) can be effectively treated during pregnancy.

Babyworld.co.uk members on vaginal discharge:

▶ *HeliG says:* 'The hospital can carry out tests to confirm whether or not the discharge is amniotic fluid, and they can offer a scan to make sure that if it is, you haven't lost too much. Amniotic fluid replaces itself anyway and I was told it would only be really serious if I felt a real gush of liquid.'

▶ *TaraM says:* 'Discharge can sometimes be quite watery, and if the loss stops, it's unlikely to be amniotic fluid. If your waters are leaking, the leakage carries on.'

● *LaraP says:* 'My friend told me she had quite heavy discharge throughout her pregnancy. Her doctor reassured her it was to keep infections from entering the uterus.'

'Knicker-watchers' of the world unite

- This affectionate term, coined by club members, stresses the importance of monitoring changes in discharge, but it shouldn't become a major concern. Remember that discharge is a normal and, in fact, necessary part of pregnancy.

- Normal hygiene should keep you feeling fresh throughout pregnancy, though if you are experiencing heavy loss, use sanitary pads. Avoid vaginal douches and scented hygiene wipes as these may cause irritation and affect the acid/alkali balance of the vagina.

- Vaginal infections are not only noticeable through the type of discharge – if you experience vaginal itching and soreness, low abdominal pain or pain during sex, consult your midwife or GP, as these may also be indicative of vaginal infections.

See also:

Thrush – page 30
Pelvic floor exercises and incontinence – page 66
Cystitis – page 68
Bleeding and spotting – page 90
First signs of labour – page 180
Babyworld.co.uk link: **www.babyworld.co.uk/faq**

"I've been having a really thick discharge and chronic itch-ing. My friend had thrush when she was pregnant, and she thinks I've got it – how can I be sure?"

THRUSH

Most of the women who've posted on this subject are clear that if you're not sure whether you have thrush, you don't have it. Itching, soreness, thick white ('cottage cheese') discharge, and stinging when passing urine are typical symptoms.

But the truth is that the only way to be sure these symptoms are due to thrush, and not to another infection, is to see your GP for a vaginal examination and for swabs to be taken. Treatment for thrush includes keeping your body cool and dry, avoiding soaps and bubble baths, avoiding scratching or rubbing and sex, and using anti-fungal medica-tion.

Creams and pessaries are safe during pregnancy – these should be obtained on prescription from your GP. Stronger oral treatments should not be used. Though the cream may not be effective, the pessary will usually clear up the problem. If your symptoms do not settle, however, see your GP for a further examination.

If a woman has vaginal thrush infection when she delivers, then there is a risk that the baby will develop thrush infection. However, thrush in a newborn baby is unlikely to be a major problem, and in most cases is easily treated.

Babyworld.co.uk members on thrush:

▶ *MagsP says:* 'There are some natural remedies, like applying natural yogurt on the affected area. Eating live yogurt too will get your intestines back to normal, as all the good bacteria will have been killed off too.'

▶ *LoriQ says:* 'If you have a vaginal delivery and you've got thrush, the baby can pick it up in the birth canal and get it in its mouth which can make it uncomfortable for the baby to breast-feed.'

▶ *Mum2B says:* 'An anti-fungal cream will help to calm the itching. Some people don't like using a pessary but it will take some time for the thrush to clear up without it. You don't have to use the applicator if you don't want to, just use your fingers instead.'

▶ *Karo says:* 'Make sure you don't use any perfumed products in the bath or shower, wear cotton underwear and keep yourself cool and dry.'

▶ *MariG says:* 'I suffered from thrush frequently, not only during pregnancy, until someone advised me to give up eating mushrooms. I did, and haven't had a bout of it since in three years.'

The low-down on thrush

Some people seem to be particularly prone to thrush, without any particular clues as to who or why. Pregnancy is known to make thrush infection more likely. Thrush is caused by yeasts which live on the skin, and in the mouth, gut, and vagina, usually without any problem. These yeasts are kept under control by bacteria, and the body's immune system. Certain conditions, such as taking antibiotics, upset the normal balance, allowing yeasts to overgrow, and result in thrush. Recurrent thrush episodes can also occasionally be an indication of diabetes, see your GP or midwife to arrange a blood test.

See also:

Vaginal discharge – page 28

Babyworld.co.uk link: **www.babyworld.co.uk/faq**

"My breasts are still really sensitive to the touch – sometimes it feels like they're going to burst! What can I do to ease the soreness?"

SWOLLEN AND SORE BREASTS

Sometimes your breasts may feel so painful that you can't bear them to be touched, or even accidentally brushed against. They may also throb or feel hot. It might be small comfort to you to know that all this is a sure sign that your breasts are getting ready to feed your baby. But that's exactly what's going on as milk-producing cells and ducts grow rapidly, and blood flow increases.

This tenderness usually eases around the middle of pregnancy. Until then make sure you're using the right size and type of bra – a good supporting bra is essential during the day. You may need to change the size of bra at regular intervals during pregnancy. At night, you might find it more comfortable to wear a sleep bra.

Later on, there may well still be further changes to your breasts, like the darkening of your nipples and areolas (the circles of skin around your nipples). You may see prominent veins running across your breasts. From mid-pregnancy onwards, you may even leak a little colostrum (early milk) – but don't worry if this doesn't happen. It's no indication of future problems with breastfeeding as the milk will come through when it's needed.

Babyworld.co.uk members on swollen and sore breasts:

▶ *Kala says:* 'My breasts are still very sore. I go to sleep lying on my side then in my sleep roll onto my tummy, and wake myself up because they are so sore."

▶ *Tiloa says:* 'I've found that using warm (not hot) heat pads and cool gel packs (you can get ones designed for breasts) really helped soothe the soreness.'

▶ *Sara71 says:* 'Whether you leak or not in pregnancy isn't thought to be an indicator of whether you can breastfeed or not. The same goes for size also, some women's breasts grow rapidly and noticeably and others grow much slower.'

▶ *Filp says:* 'If you're at all concerned about anything to do with your breasts, get it checked out by your GP. If you have a red, scaly rash going from the nipple to the areola, any lumps or puckering get it checked out. Just because you are pregnant does not mean you don't have to check your breasts regularly. Most lumps and bumps are nothing to worry about.'

▶ *Mags01 says:* 'Last time I was pregnant I wore a sports bra in bed for extra support, I haven't got to that stage yet, but no doubt that's still to come.'

▶ *Suse says:* 'I was told to stuff cold cabbage leaves down my bra after I gave birth and I've been beginning to wonder if it would work. I might give it a go!'

▶ *Hanna5 says:* 'The soreness should pass, but in the meantime wearing a supportive bra often helps. If your breasts feel hot, try putting a cold flannel, or a bag of frozen peas against them (less of an option in bed, of course). Sometimes gentle massage can help, and some women find that cutting out caffeine helps too.'

See also:
Breast sensitivity and other early signs – page 10
Itching and obstetric cholestasis – page 110
Babyworld.co.uk link: **www.babyworld.co.uk/faq**

"I'm so exhausted all the time I can barely function – when will this overwhelming tiredness ease, and what can I do to control it?"

TIREDNESS

Tiredness can cause real problems for women in the first and last trimesters. In the early stages, you may feel excessively tired and lethargic. This is caused by pregnancy hormones.

Rest is the most effective remedy, though it is often easier said than done, especially if you're working or looking after young children. You can help to boost your energy levels by eating regular, balanced meals. This is also the time to get your partner, family and friends to help out with things like shopping, chores around the house and cooking.

Towards the end of pregnancy, tiredness is normally due to increased size and weight, because your system is working extra hard to support you and your baby, and because you may not be sleeping very well at night. If you are particularly affected by nausea or heartburn, and not eating as a consequence, you will start to feel more tired.

Tiredness is often worse for women who are overweight, or who are pregnant with more than one child. Severe tiredness may also be a sign that you have anaemia, so it may be worth getting your iron levels checked by your GP or midwife.

Babyworld.co.uk members on tiredness:

▶ *Angi says:* 'This is very, very common in the early weeks of pregnancy. Growing a baby is hard work for your body, and also pregnancy hormones have a kind of sedative effect. This overwhelming tiredness does usually pass once you get into the second three months, though.'

▶ *Kar2 says:* 'Dried apricots are good for an energy boost as they are high in natural sugar and iron. They taste pretty good too!'

▶ *LoriP says:* 'I have actually found that I feel 100 per cent better if I can drag myself out for a swim. I know it sounds a bit far fetched, but it always works for me.'

▶ *JenaL says:* 'The tiredness of early pregnancy is to a large extent hormonal, so actually there isn't a lot you can do to boost your energy levels, but complex carbohydrates (whole grains, oats, pasta, rice etc) might sustain you for longer, and have the advantage of being fairly bland.'

▶ *Sammo says:* 'I really do think that tiredness is related to my sickness. The more tired I am the worse I feel – I have had lots of sleep over the weekend and I feel fine.'

▶ *Marthasmum says:* 'I am sleeping between client appointments in the day because I literally cannot stay awake and function otherwise. It is a tiredness that is as overwhelming when I wake up in the morning as it is when I go to bed at night! I have been recommended exercise but a 30 minute walk is enough to tire me out completely. It is meant to energise... I'm sure that will be the case further into the pregnancy.'

▶ *Kato says:* 'I started checking what I could eat that contained lots of iron. Some cereals have up to 48 per cent of the recommended daily amounts. I've been having a bowl in the morning for about two weeks, and I feel a little less tired.'

See also:
Anaemia – page 36
Insomnia – page 78
Blooming and boosted energy – page 80
Keeping fit and exercising – page 120
Babyworld.co.uk link: **www.babyworld.co.uk/faq**

> **"I've been told I'm suffering from anaemia, what causes it and are there any alternatives to taking iron tablets?"**

ANAEMIA

Midwife says: If you have anaemia, it means that the level of haemoglobin in your blood is low. Haemoglobin is a substance in your red blood cells that carries oxygen round your body. In order to produce haemoglobin, your body needs various things, including folic acid and iron. The most common cause of anaemia in pregnancy is not having enough iron, particularly in the last three months, when the baby's iron needs increase. Anaemia can lead to your feeling tired and washed out, as well as dizzy and breathless, so if you're experiencing these symptoms, it's wise to let your midwife know.

What actually constitutes anaemia in pregnancy is a matter of some debate. This is because it's normal for your haemoglobin levels to be lower when you're pregnant, because the volume of the liquid part of your blood increases, so your blood is relatively 'thinner'. This is thought to aid blood flow through the placenta. The debate is over how much lower is normal. The usual treatment for anaemia is taking iron tablets, to boost haemoglobin production, but there are differences of opinion among doctors and midwives over the haemoglobin levels at which these should be prescribed. One of the disadvantages of taking them is that they can cause constipation or diarrhoea or sickness. Eating an iron-rich diet can also help to boost your iron levels.

If you have severe anaemia, which is rare, or it doesn't improve after taking iron tablets for a while, further blood tests would be likely to be offered to find out the cause of the problem and establish the most appropriate treatment.

Babyworld.co.uk members on anaemia:

▶ *Tizz says:* 'Liquid iron tends to be better tolerated and absorbed. Doctors tend to prescribe tablets which are very cheap but do affect your bowels and can cause stomach pain. Plus they are less well absorbed.'

▶ *Pip180 says:* 'You can see either your midwife or doctor and they will take some blood and send it off to check your iron levels. Try in the meantime to eat more iron rich foods such as leafy green vegetables, red meat, baked beans, cereal etc.'

▶ *Marthasmum says:* 'If the iron tablets make you constipated, dried apricots are good for both that and are also a source of iron. Try to drink fresh orange with your meals and cut down on your tea intake.'

▶ *Tico says:* 'I've been taking a pregnancy multi vitamin tablet and eating more high iron foods along with vitamin C, which aids iron absorption. Don't drink tea when you eat, it stops the uptake of iron. Also, the iron in meat is absorbed five times better than veggie-based iron.'

▶ *Sali says:* 'I didn't want to take tablets so have been using natural iron sachets called spatone. It seems to be pretty gentle and you just put it in a glass of orange juice to aid absorption.'

▶ *Peta says:* 'I asked my midwife about this and she said that if you keep taking folic acid throughout pregnancy, it can help your body to retain iron.'

See also:
Fainting – page 38
Constipation – page 44
Babyworld.co.uk link: **www.babyworld.co.uk/faq**

"I fainted in the queue at the post office the other day – it was so scary. What caused it and how can I stop it happening again?"

FAINTING AND DIZZINESS

Dizziness is very common in pregnancy, and is due mainly to the effects of pregnancy hormones which cause widening of blood vessels. You can't really predict when you'll feel dizzy or faint, but there are things you can do, and avoid, which will reduce the risks of fainting.

Standing for a lengthy period leads to pooling of the blood in the dilated veins, so that dizziness or fainting is a risk – so find someone else to do the ironing and make sure you insist on your right to a seat on the train or bus. If you do find yourself standing around, try to move about and exercise your feet and legs.

Some women feel faint when they stand up suddenly. Try to stand up in a slow, flowing movement and if you do feel faint, sit down again and take deep breaths as rapidly as possible. Hot baths cause the blood vessels to dilate even further so get out very slowly while holding onto something.

Fainting is unpleasant and disorientating, but rest assured that you will come round quickly and that fainting is not a danger in itself to you or your baby.

Dizzy spells can sometimes be linked to low blood sugar, so it's best to eat regular light meals. Sustained dizziness may be linked to anaemia, so if you're worried it may be a good idea to get your iron levels checked.

Babyworld.co.uk members on fainting:

▶ *SuziM says:* 'I was standing on the train as there were no seats and suddenly felt really sick and dizzy and had to sit down on the floor! I think it was because I hadn't eaten anything for a while.'

▶ *Kato says:* 'I have had the occasional dizzy spell when making beds and cleaning bathrooms as a result of repeatedly bending down and getting up. Not eating breakfast sometimes before I get on with these jobs probably aggravates it for me.'

▶ *TeriP says:* 'When the nurse tries to take my blood, I come over hot and faint and then start seeing what I can only describe as black rain falling then everything sounds like I am in a long tunnel. My husband has to come with me to distract me while they try and take my blood.'

▶ *Pip180 says:* 'As you get bigger, the weight of the uterus affects the blood flow in your arteries and can cause fainting and low blood pressure.'

▶ *Gio says:* 'The minute I feel even remotely dizzy I sit down – regardless of where I am – and tip my head as far down between my legs as I can manage.'

▶ *Tula says:* 'I make a point of always endeavouring to have someone with me if I know I'm going to be out and about and on my feet for a while, or if I'm going somewhere 'remote' without many people about just in case I have a turn. This can be a pain at times because you end up feeling a bit of a dependent invalid but it's preferable to the alternative of coming unstuck and being alone!'

▶ *Marthasmum says:* 'My midwife told me that my blood pressure is low so I should take care when standing for long periods of time and be careful not to move quickly because it will make me feel faint or dizzy.'

See also:
Anaemia – page 36
Babyworld.co.uk link: **www.babyworld.co.uk/faq**

> **"I thought pregnant women were supposed to glow – all I've got is a load of spots and greasy skin. What am I doing wrong?"**

SPOTS

Whatever your age, profession or level of maturity, pregnancy can be a great leveller. For some women this means a return to the awkward teenage phase of spots and oily skin. There's no way to second-guess the phenomenon, as pregnancy hormones affect different women in totally different ways. Some may be left with unblemished, radiant skin throughout pregnancy, and some may find, as one of the antenatal club members puts it, that they 'wake up one morning as a pepperoni pizza'.

Unfortunately most of the standard spot treatments are unsafe for use in pregnancy, though there are some safe, natural washes and creams available – consult your pharmacist for advice. If all else fails, take comfort from the fact that skin is generally healthier and clearer in the second half of pregnancy.

Babyworld.co.uk members on spots:

▶ *Teri says:* 'I have spots breaking out on my chest. I use Tea tree products and wash at lunchtime in work to keep my skin fresh.'

Han67 says:

▶ 'My skin clears up during pregnancy! If only I could bottle the hormone then I could enjoy pristine skin all the time!'

▶ *Ozz says:* 'I've always suffered from awfully oily skin and lots of pimples. It's really got me down at times, but since getting pregnant my skin has been glowing. I think it's the progesterone surge!'

▶ *Suse says:* 'Tea tree oil is very good as it's naturally antiseptic. You could also try using face packs on a regular basis.'

▶ *Lori says:* I have got zillions of spots. I'm so self conscious about them that I have a permanent orange face from all the make-up I am wearing.'

▶ *Zed34 says:* 'I know it sounds weird, but a dab of toothpaste always clears my spots up. Put it on before bed.'

▶ *Tula says:* 'The doctor told me that pregnancy would be the best thing for my skin as it would sort my hormones out for me. Well, for the first eight weeks my skin was radiant, not a spot in sight. Now, however, it's a different story. My shoulders, chest, back, neck and around my hairline are so greasy and I'm getting lots of horrid pimples.'

▶ *Mum2B says:* 'It is not easy to predict how your skin is going to react. Keep your skin care routine as basic as possible and use a plain moisturiser to minimise problems.'

The skin you're in

Spots aren't the only skin changes you may notice in pregnancy. Changes in pigmentation are extremely common, affecting 90 per cent of women. You may notice the following:

● darkening of the area around your nipples
● a brown line down the centre of your stomach (linea nigra)
● darkening of freckles, moles or birthmarks
● brown patches on your face (worsened by exposure to the sun)

While you should always monitor changes to your skin, and consult your doctor about any moles which change in size or are sore or cracked, the changes listed above are all perfectly natural in pregnancy, and will usually fade completely once your baby is born.

See also:

Babyworld.co.uk link: **www.babyworld.co.uk/faq**

"Right now it seems like I'm either incredibly excited or really down – is this what they mean by mood swings – my poor partner doesn't know where he stands any more!"

MOOD SWINGS

Blame those hormones. High progesterone levels (during pregnancy or before periods) do cause mood swings for many women – though not all. However, it's also important to acknowledge that pregnancy is a time of enormous change – physically, emotionally, socially and financially. It takes time to adjust to these changes and they can be overwhelming. Bursting into tears or raging at the world doesn't mean that there is anything wrong with you or your baby. It is just a way of coping with an exciting, frightening, amazing time in your life. As long as the lows are balanced by highs there is nothing to worry about.

If you do feel despairing or unable to cope, try talking to your midwife or doctor about this. Some women become clinically depressed during pregnancy and there is support and treatment available. If there are specific things in your life that make you unhappy and anxious, now is the time to tackle them, before your baby is born.

Babyworld.co.uk members on mood swings:

▶ *Peri says:* 'I don't think I realised that my mood swings were related to the pregnancy until the final trimester, when it occurred to me that all those hormonal changes must have an effect on mood. I also think it's related to the anxieties about such a huge life change too, though. Having our first child is probably the biggest thing many of us ever do, and the fears and worries can be overwhelming.'

▶ *Marthasmum says:* 'There are definitely times that the smallest thing can set you off. I remember being startled at how emotionally involved I became with some TV plot lines, news stories or incidents in books.'

▶ *Mum2B says:* 'I was more depressed first and second trimesters and I feel it's just adjusting to the thing growing inside you. Zapping your energy, depriving you of sleep and also providing a nice list of doubts – everything from giving birth and hospital bag to whether you and your partner are going to be OK.'

▶ *Gio says:* 'I think stress has a big part to play as well. I overdid it for a fortnight at work, and the weekend following this I was a mess. I felt like a possessed woman, picking fights with my partner and then not wanting him to be too far away from me. Crying uncontrollably for half an hour and then being fine. Very weird.'

▶ *Kato says:* 'I feel a bit left out. I don't know why, but I am not going through any mood swings at all. I cry really easily – at adverts on TV and stuff, but I am generally much happier I think. I have an inner calm which I never had before.'

▶ *Maj says:* 'The key is to try and relax. I'm working ten hour days but try to take an hour in the afternoon to get away from my desk for a bit of peace and quiet. I'm also trying not to arrange too many things for after work – quiet nights in and lots of sleep *really* have helped me.'

▶ *Sala says:* 'I just take the dogs for a walk or have a bath when I feel myself boiling over.'

▶ *Mio says:* 'I know from experience that when someone gives you that 'hormonal' speech you just want to smack them, hormones or not! Sometimes all you need is to go off and have a good cry, or rant and rave to get it off your chest, and I'm sure every one of us has felt like that.'

See also:

Feeling anxious – page 18
Babyworld.co.uk link: **www.babyworld.co.uk/faq**

"My bowels have been blocked for days and I'm feeling really sluggish. What can I do to get more regular?"

CONSTIPATION

As far as bowel movements go, pregnancy seems to be a case of feast or famine. And the latter is more common, with constipation causing serious discomfort for many women throughout. It's not helped by the fact that certain other pregnancy treatments – especially iron tablets for anaemia – can exacerbate constipation.

It's hard to completely eradicate constipation but there are plenty of ways to help keep your bowels happy which are perfectly safe to try in pregnancy. Among the most common are eating more fresh fruit and vegetables, drinking plenty of water, and keeping active. Walking, swimming, and yoga all help your digestive process.

So the trick for 'keeping regular' is to be regular in your habits. Drink at least eight glasses of water a day. Take a brisk walk for twenty minutes daily to stimulate your bowels. You don't necessarily need a high-fibre diet: a few dried prunes or apricots may be all you need each day to help your constipation, or there is a healthfood product called 'Golden Linseed' which can help get you going. If all the above fails, then your GP may prescribe you lactulose which is a sugar-based laxative, designed to soften the motion and make it easier to pass.

Babyworld.co.uk members on constipation:

▶ *JP says:* 'I took flaxseed oil in my first pregnancy and have been taking it before conception this time around. It not only completely eases constipation but is an essential oil for the baby's brain and eye development.'

▶ *Sharl says:* 'For some women iron tablets give them constipation and others get the runs. Have you tried taking it every other day to see if that helps?'

▶ *Tizz says:* 'I have coeliac disease (gluten-free diet needed) so most of the recommended foods are a no-no for me. I'm finding that jacket potatoes smothered in baked beans are helping. Grapes are good too.'

▶ *Han67 says:* 'Eat well to the last – I had constipation while in labour (thanks to iron tablets) and it gave me excruciating back-ache on top of everything else.'

▶ *Loz says:* 'I find that Weetabix and orange juice does the trick for me. But not together!'

▶ *Teri says:* 'Prunes and grapes are great, as is any type of dried fruit. It's also really important to drink loads of water as dehydration is the number one reason for constipation.'

▶ *Tula says:* 'Liquorice can ease constipation. It is OK to eat in moderation as part of a healthy and varied diet. There is a substance in liquorice called glycyrrhizin, and I've heard that if this is eaten in large quantities it may be linked to premature or earlier labour.'

See also:
Heartburn – page 24
Anaemia – page 36
Haemorrhoids – page 46
Flatulence – page 48
Keeping fit and exercising – page 120
Babyworld.co.uk link: **www.babyworld.co.uk/faq**

> **"I've got agonising sore lumps on my bottom. Are these piles? If so, how can I get rid of them?"**

HAEMORRHOIDS (PILES)

Haemorrhoids are common throughout pregnancy, and can frequently cause irritation and bleeding. They're often a side-effect of constipation, so your chances of avoiding them are improved by keeping your digestive system healthy with a good diet of lots of fresh fruit and vegetables, drinking plenty of water and exercising regularly.

If you do develop piles, they will usually settle fairly quickly after delivery, although they won't disappear completely and might recur in future pregnancies. Steroid-containing ointments may be used, though not for prolonged periods of time. If these are applied regularly over a week they can lead to dramatic improvements.

Babyworld.co.uk members on piles:

▶ *KayM says:* 'Treatments like Anusol can help with piles, and also holding a small packet of frozen peas against your back passage might help to shrink them.'

▶ *Marthasmum says:* 'With my piles, everyone was saying use an ice pack, but I used a hot water bottle which was much better.'

▶ *Kari says:* 'My doctor gave me steroid cream and told me to take cold baths and use an ice pack.'

▶ *Pip180 says:* 'Fybogel is fine for pregnancy. I used to get it on prescription – along with piles suppositories and indigestion liquid – oh, the glamour!'

▶ *Teri says:* 'Pain in your rear may be the start of piles or it could be something called proctalgia, which can occur if you are constipated. It is like an intense spasm of the muscles in that area and it *really* hurts.'

▶ *Suki says:* 'Apparently witch hazel on a tissue held between your cheeks can be quite effective.'

▶ *Suse says:* 'I had it bad both times at the end of pregnancy and after the birth. My midwife said don't give birth lying on your back as this doesn't help – always give birth on all fours!'

See also:
Constipation – page 44
Keeping fit and exercising – page 120
Babyworld.co.uk link: **www.babyworld.co.uk/faq**

> **"I've started to suffer really badly with wind. It's really embarrassing – and quite uncomfortable too."**

FLATULENCE

Just when you thought it was safe to go back in the water…pregnancy produces another dignity-stripping side-effect that's hard to explain away. Unless you have a dog, of course.

Excess wind is a direct result of the presence of pregnancy hormones progesterone and relaxin. They act particularly on 'smooth' muscle (like that in the walls of our gut) to relax and loosen it. Though this increases the flow of blood to the baby and loosens the joints of the pelvis ready for birth, it also causes a sluggish gut – leading to indigestion, nausea, heartburn, constipation and wind.

As soon as your baby is born you'll get back to normal, but until then try to eat high fibre carbohydrate food – wholegrain bread, jacket potatoes, rice and so on. These can help the action of the gut. Eat five portions of fruit and vegetables each day, and drink at least eight glasses of water. For obvious reasons, try to avoid beans and lentils, eggs, and cabbage-type vegetables.

Exercise can also help – especially swimming, brisk walking and yoga. Activity of any kind promotes healthy digestion.

Babyworld.co.uk members on flatulence:

▶ *Peta says:* 'Avoid eating fruit at the end of a meal – try it at the start instead, or on an empty stomach. It produces lots more gas, which gets trapped if it has to wait for the other food to digest first!'

▶ *Pip180 says:* 'A bowl of All bran every morning sorts me out! It constantly feels like my guts are churning round! Fortunately my husband uses my gastro-intestinal misfortune as a source of humour, and delights in asking 'was that you?' every time the sink gurgles.'

▶ *KP says:* 'My kids think it is hilarious, I can also burp like a rugby player now too.'

▶ *Joele says:* 'Windy feelings are likely to be a result either of pressure on your bowel, or due to the effects of pregnancy hormones on your gut.'

▶ *Suki says:* 'I suffered badly with wind in the first 12 weeks. I think it's the increase in your progesterone levels (I was on progesterone supplements for first 12 weeks) but now since I stopped them I seem to be a lot better.'

▶ *MelP says:* 'If you find you have a lot of trapped gas in your stomach try sitting forward and leaning slightly to your left as this will allow the gas to gather at the top of your stomach – then you can release it in a most unladylike way!'

See also:
Heartburn – page 24
Constipation – page 44
Smoking, drinking and drugs – page 118
Keeping fit and exercising – page 120
Babyworld.co.uk link: **www.babyworld.co.uk /faq**

"What's happening to my mouth and teeth? – my gums seem to bleed loads, but I struggle to brush my teeth because the sensation makes me ill. Help!"

TOOTHCARE AND BLEEDING GUMS

A double whammy of increased blood supply and pregnancy hormones can make your gums very soft and spongy. They may bleed when you brush your teeth, or eat something hard like an apple. But if nausea is making it harder to clean your teeth, pieces of food may get trapped in your gums, and this may cause infection. Severe gum infection can cause pregnancy problems as the germs travel around your body.

There's no magic solution, it's simply a case of trying different methods to see what works for you. The first step is to tackle the nausea – perhaps by trying a different toothpaste, bland children's varieties are sometimes better, or by swapping your toothbrush for a cotton bud or just by rubbing toothpaste on with the tip of your finger until the nausea subsides.

Other alternatives to brushing include swilling with mouthwash (which is safe to use during pregnancy), and may also help to treat gum problems, and sugar-free chewing gum. Neither of these is ideal as a replacement to brushing, but in the short term they are better than nothing.

An alternative approach is to think about which foods would be good to eat at the times when you cannot clean your teeth. Avoid sugary foods like biscuits and acidic fruits like apples late at night, go for celery or a carrot instead. These will help to clean between your teeth and around your gums and they'll get the saliva flowing too. If you're still stuck for options, speak to the dental hygienist attached to your dentist's practice. As with most of the problems exacerbated by hormonal changes, your gums should get back to normal soon after your baby's birth.

Babyworld.co.uk members on bleeding gums:

▶ *Kara says:* 'See your dentist now that it is free for a check-up, and maybe try a softer toothbrush.'

▶ *Gio says:* 'There's an antiseptic mouthwash called Corsodyl which is for bleeding gums, and it's fine for use in pregnancy. It can temporarily stain your teeth, though, so don't have tea or coffee just after using it!'

Babyworld.co.uk members on brushing:

▶ *Suki7 says:* 'To get to your back teeth, scrape your nail along the tooth surface, especially where it meets the gum and this will get off most of the plaque. As you are entitled to free dental treatment whilst pregnant, try and get an appointment for a check up and a scale and polish.'

▶ *TaraM says:* 'Brushing my teeth starts me gagging. I've found that saying 'aaaah' loudly while doing the back teeth makes it better – it's strange but true!'

▶ *Suse says:* 'I brush my teeth the best I can in the morning and evening and then chew some teeth whitening gum during the day.'

Babyworld.co.uk members on dental care:

▶ *Petal says:* 'Some dentists only do some work privately, regardless of whether you are entitled to it for free. This tends to include bridges, crowns, dentures and mouth guards. Find out whether this applies at your dental practice. The things you should definitely NOT have to pay for are checkups, scale and polishes (only two a year), extractions and fillings. It isn't recommended you have any fillings done whilst pregnant except for temporary ones.'

See also:

Morning sickness and nausea – page 20

Babyworld.co.uk link: **www.babyworld.co.uk/faq**

> **"I've started to get terrible blocked noses, and when I blow there's sometimes blood on the tissue – is this normal and how can I ease it?"**

NASAL PROBLEMS

Common nasal problems during pregnancy include stuffiness, a runny nose, and nosebleeds. These problems may start early on and can continue throughout.

The blame lies with pregnancy hormones which cause the lining of your nose and sinuses to swell, so you feel continually blocked up and stuffy. Hormones are also at fault for the widening of the tiny blood vessels in your nose, a change that increases the chance of nosebleeds. This enhanced blood supply may also cause increased mucus production, so your nose is always runny. Nice, eh?

Swelling in the sinuses can sometimes cause pain in your cheeks and behind your eyes, and may contribute to headaches. Nasal problems usually resolve themselves soon after the birth.

Babyworld.co.uk members on nasal congestion:

▶ *Pip180 says:* 'I think that the only thing you can try is saline drops or saline nose spray to try and ease the congestion.'

▶ *Mands says:* 'If you get dry or cracked lips, this might be caused by your swollen or blocked nose, especially if you're breathing with your mouth open at night.'

Nose news is good news

- **Blocked nose**: Try a steam inhalation, and put a few drops of tea tree oil in the water.

- **Breathing through your mouth at night**: Keep a glass of water handy for when you wake and use Vaseline to keep your lips moist. You may start to snore. Sleeping on your side may ease this.

- **Nosebleed**: Lean forward, pinching the sides of your nose firmly together just below the bone. Do this for at least 10 minutes.

- **Warning signs**: If you have more than two bad nosebleeds (or lots of little ones), consult your GP. Severe nosebleeds may contribute to anaemia, or may be a sign of underlying illness.

Sometimes stuffiness and a runny nose can be linked to sensitivities and allergies. Most medicinal hay fever treatments like antihistamines should not be used in pregnancy, though some are allowed – always consult your GP for more advice first. There are herbal, homeopathic and natural treatments available – again, you should consult a qualified practitioner before taking any in pregnancy.

Babyworld.co.uk members on hayfever and allergies:

▶ *Peri says:* 'Hay fever treatments that some people find helpful include eating locally produced honey, and putting some Vaseline around your nostrils, to prevent you from breathing pollen in.'

▶ *SamF says:* 'I usually take Beconase. This is a topical steroid in the form of a nasal spray. It works quickly and, I find, can be very effective when my hayfever is not too bad. My doctor told me that Beconase and similar topical steroid sprays are OK to use, particularly later on during pregnancy.'

▶ *Kato says:* 'I swear by green tea and homeopathic tissue salts. I am very, very loath to give either up – because one of them seems to be having an effect!'

See also:
Trying alternative remedies – page 136
Babyworld.co.uk link: **www.babyworld.co.uk/faq**

"I woke up last night in agony, with a sharp pain in my lower leg. It still feels a bit bruised. What caused this, and what can I do to prevent it?"

CRAMP

Cramp in the calves is common in pregnancy and isn't usually a sign of anything sinister. You might also feel 'bruised' for a day or so afterwards.

If you cannot relieve the pain by stretching the muscle or walking around, it is worth speaking to your midwife – there is a small possibility that the pain could be from DVT (deep vein thrombosis), which is very rare, but is also a serious problem if left unchecked.

There is no specific preventative for cramp. Some women find that drinking a milky drink before bed helps, while others recommend drinking tonic water.

Babyworld.co.uk members on cramp:

▶ *LoriP says:* 'I suffered from cramps a lot. I read that it might be down to a potassium deficiency. I drank a glass of milk each night before bed, as apparently the calcium helps absorb potassium more easily – perhaps try a banana with it too. I didn't suffer with them after that.'

▶ *Tami says:* 'The best way to cure the cramp is to straighten out your leg and then pull your foot up towards your knee. It hurts to do it but it stops the cramp almost immediately. I suffered from cramp with my last pregnancy, but this works brilliantly.'

▶ *Pip180 says:* 'There's not all that much you can do to prevent cramp, though doing some feet exercises (pointing your toes up, not down, and circling your feet in both directions) for a few minutes before you go to bed might help. If you relax as much as you can when you get a cramp, that might help it to pass more quickly.'

▶ *Mum2B says:* 'I was getting cramps because I was dehydrated. So I started drinking at least two litres of water after 4pm (and I hate water) but they have stopped!'

▶ *Jups says:* 'The best thing to do is to stand up then stretch the muscle by pushing against a wall with the offending leg straight out behind you and the other leg bent. It will hurt but it is the only way to stop the cramp.'

▶ *Mia says:* 'Leg cramps are quite common in pregnancy. They can feel quite bruised for a day or so afterwards. Some people swear by bananas for potassium, Greek yoghurt for calcium, tonic water for quinine or crisps for salt.'

▶ *Sash78 says:* 'I don't suffer cramp often, but if I wake up with it the odd time I always take deep breaths in and out to relax and it subsides quickly.'

See also:
Babyworld.co.uk link: **www.babyworld.co.uk/faq**

"I really don't want stretch marks – what's the best way to avoid them?"

STRETCH MARKS

The first cosmetics company that perfects a cream, oil or gel that is guaranteed to combat stretch marks will have a licence to print money – as well as the undying love of women the world over. Unfortunately, until then, we have to accept the fact that stretch marks are an inevitability for some women and that no amount of massage and moisturising can lessen the impact.

For many women, stretch marks come as a result of hormonal changes that weaken the skin, allowing skin fibres to tear. The thin, red streaks can appear on breasts, thighs, bottoms and bellies but they do fade to a pale silvery colour in time, and, depending on your skin tone, they might become almost unnoticeable.

Babyworld.co.uk members on stretch marks:

▶ *KyraD says:* 'It's a bit of a myth that stretch marks can be prevented. Some people get them and some don't, despite what you put on them. This being my third pregnancy, I've pretty much given up...especially as they fade afterwards anyway.'

▶ *Olli says:* 'If you are going to get stretch marks there isn't anything you can do, but rubbing in the cream helps you get used to your bigger body, and you can talk to the baby while you do it.'

▶ *Melrose says:* 'Whether you get stretch marks depends on the structure of your skin, so there isn't really anything you can do to prevent them, I'm afraid.'

▶ *Zenna says:* 'I give my bump a lovely rub with baby oil gel at bedtime to send it to sleep. I started using this as my tummy got really dry after my holidays – and cocoa butter was making me gag!'

Scratching the itch

A knock-on problem arising from stretch marks is that they can become irritated and itchy. Given that stretch marks can appear from as early as three to four months, that's a long time to resist the urge to have a good scratch. Here's a couple of handy tips from club members:

▶ *LoisF says:* 'You can get calamine cream from the chemist, which is worth using on stretch marks as it is also moisturising. If that doesn't help you can speak to your GP or pharmacist to see if you could take any anti-histamines to reduce the itch.'

▶ *Hari says:* 'It's not the most comfortable thing to try but ice in a tea towel has worked well for me. I sit watching TV like that and the tickling feeling wears off eventually! I think it just numbs the skin a bit. One warning though, it makes my baby very active!'

While itchy stretch marks are common and rarely a cause for concern, localised itching, particularly on the palms of your hands and soles of your feet, may be a sign of a more serious condition called obstetric cholestasis. Speak to your GP or midwife if you have any concerns about localised itching.

See also:

Itching and obstetric cholestasis – page 110
Your changing appearance – page 116
Babyworld.co.uk link: **www.babyworld.co.uk/faq**

> **"I love my legs, so I'm really keen to avoid varicose veins if I can – what should I do to steer clear of them?"**

VARICOSE VEINS

Whether or not you get varicose veins in pregnancy may be more a question of your genetic make-up than any other factor. If your mother or sisters had varicose veins, you are more likely than other women to suffer.

Even so, there's still some tried-and-tested remedies to ease the seriousness of varicose veins. Eating a balanced diet with plenty of fruit and vegetables and avoiding too much high-fat or sugary food will keep excess weight off your legs. Some people reckon that eating raw onions, garlic and parsley may help combat varicose veins by boosting the circulation – if not the social life. Regular exercise – especially brisk walking, swimming and dancing – helps strengthen your heart and lungs, and tones your muscles.

On a day-to-day basis it's vital to keep your legs moving whilst standing still, by 'walking on the spot' or standing on tiptoes at regular intervals. If you're stuck behind a desk at work wriggle your feet, circling the ankles, and flexing the ankle joints. Avoid clothes that restrict circulation to your lower legs. Think seriously about wearing support tights. When resting, lie on your side with your head on one pillow and your legs raised on two or three more.

Some women suffer from extremely painful vulval varicose veins. These can sometimes cause problems with the birth, depending on how bad they are, and where they are located. On rare occasions, they may be so serious that an elective caesarean section is recommended following examination by an obstetrician late in pregnancy.

Babyworld.co.uk members on varicose veins:

▶ *Kato says:* 'My friend suffers from varicose veins and has a covering make-up she puts on her legs if she wants to wear anything short.'

▶ *Mum2B says:* 'In my last pregnancy I had a prominent vein on my left shin – I can still see where it was, but it went down after the baby was born. This time round the other leg is suffering. I think it's been damaged by driving and/or crossing my legs as that is when it aches the most.'

▶ *Skiff says:* 'I have the very uncomfortable vulval varicose veins. They feel very heavy and make bowel movements quite difficult too, much in the same way that haemorrhoids do. Resting is the only effective way of reducing the swelling, although tight pants, paracetamol and cold compresses do have some effect.'

Han67 says: 'Varicose veins run in the family normally (so I'm seriously worried) but I have heard that wearing support tights can help.'

▶ *Peta says:* 'I have never had varicose veins before and the bottom half of my legs are purple (hundreds of tiny veins). My midwife said it's all very normal and should go once the baby is born – it's because of all the extra blood in the body.'

See also:
Your changing appearance – page 116
Keeping fit and exercising – page 120
Babyworld.co.uk link: **www.babyworld.co.uk/faq**

"I've been getting nasty pains in my ribs when I sit on the sofa at the end of the day. What's causing this and how can it be treated?"

RIB PAIN AND STITCHES

Pregnancy hormones can cause softening of ligaments throughout the body and this makes women more prone to pain coming from the skeleton and its muscles and joints.

Pain in the lower ribs is common in the later stages of pregnancy, particularly the last three months, when the uterus is enlarging and starting to compress the ribs. This pain tends to be worse when sitting and easier when standing or lying down. It will ease off when the baby's head engages in the pelvis or at the onset of labour.

It's unlikely that there's a serious cause for this pain, but it's a good idea to see your GP to try to establish what the cause is and to rule out other causes of chest and rib pain, such as a chest infection.

You can ease the pain by taking extra care with your posture – try to stand up straight and sit in a good position with support for your lower back. Lying on your side when sleeping may also help to alleviate rib pain. Swimming is beneficial, especially backstroke, so it would be a good thing to try, as it is the sort of activity you can continue throughout pregnancy.

Another potential factor in rib pain that's worth bearing in mind is the position and movement of your baby – it's quite common for a baby to 'pummel' the rib area, or to become wedged in an uncomfortable spot, causing pressure and pain.

Babyworld.co.uk members on rib pain:

▶ *Mel02 says:* 'Try to sit and stand as upright as possible to lift your ribs off your uterus. Putting your hands in the air might give some temporary relief, and another temporary measure is kneeling forwards over a pile of pillows, or a beanbag or birthing ball if you have one, with your hands above your head. Rib pain usually eases when your baby starts moving down into your pelvis.'

▶ *CaitlinJ says:* 'I was getting really kicked by my baby during the day in my rib area but I noticed it was only happening when I wore something with a slightly tighter waistband. It's worth trying some looser clothing for a few days to see if that helps.

A stitch in time

- Stitch-like pains are common for many women, and while there are several explanations, the cause is very rarely serious. If your baby is moving well, the problem is likely to be attributed to pain from the two ligaments, one each side, that go from the top of the uterus into the groin, to hold the uterus in place. As the uterus gets bigger, these ligaments stretch and this can sometimes lead to pain, especially if there's any extra strain on them from walking, getting out of a chair, lifting or bending, or even coughing and sneezing.

- Of course, just because they aren't serious, they can still be painful and if you experience frequent or prolonged pain, you can be referred to a physiotherapist for treatment. For any severe abdominal pain that's constant, and is associated with the baby not moving, you should seek urgent medical advice.

See also:

Feeling the baby move – page 82
Babyworld.co.uk link: **www.babyworld.co.uk/faq**

"I got home from work today and my ankles are like tree trunks. They're so swollen I can barely put on my shoes. What's causing this?"

SWOLLEN ANKLES, HANDS AND FINGERS

It's very common for women to retain extra fluid while pregnant. The fluid is needed to help soften up the body so that it gives as the baby grows. It also helps to prepare the pelvic joints and tissues for opening up to allow the baby to be delivered.

About a quarter of the weight women gain during pregnancy is retained fluid. Some of this extra fluid tends to collect in the feet, ankles and hands, causing swelling (oedema) and puffiness, especially in the later stages of pregnancy. You may start to notice swelling from around five months. It's more of a problem for women who are overweight, or who gain a lot of weight during pregnancy, or who are pregnant with more than one baby. It can be worse at the end of the day or if you have been standing for a long time, or in hot weather.

Slight swelling isn't a problem, although it can be uncomfortable, and also inconvenient if you find that your shoes no longer fit and your rings are too tight. But if you notice any sudden swelling in your hands and your face, let your midwife or doctor know straight away. It could be a sign of pre-eclampsia.

Babyworld.co.uk members on swelling:

▶ *Mags01 says:* 'I started to experience swelling at about 20 weeks. The suggestions I have been given to try to alleviate it are to drink loads of water and to rest with my feet up as much as possible. I get my husband to massage my feet, ankles and calves in an upward direction. It helps to get the circulation going and move the fluid a bit.'

▶ *Suse says:* 'I've got swollen fingers and my ankles are puffy too. I saw my midwife yesterday to get my blood pressure checked and she said it was nothing to worry about. Worth getting yours checked though if it is worrying you.'

▶ *Kari says:* 'The only thing I can suggest is resting with your feet elevated whenever you can, it seems to ease the swelling in my feet if I do that.'

▶ *Coel says:* 'If you're suffering at work, you could always turn a bin upside down and put pillows on top to sit with your legs up, I've moved my PC and desk around so that I can sit with my feet up.'

▶ *MayaP says:* 'I'd suggest wearing support tights and trying to rotate your ankles regularly as well.'

▶ *Suki says:* 'My ankles are only swelling when I've done a lot of walking or if it is too hot. If you can lie with your feet up against the wall for five minutes or so, it does help.'

Some swell ideas

- Wear low-heeled shoes
- Wear support tights or stockings
- Don't wear clothes that are tight round your ankles or wrists
- Press cooled dark green cabbage leaves to your ankles and feet (honest!)
- If your fingers are swelling, take your rings off before they get stuck

See also:

Pre-eclampsia – page 106
Babyworld.co.uk link: **www.babyworld.co.uk/faq**

"After a long day at work I get terrible backache – is this
normal in pregnancy and what are the safe treatments?"

BACKACHE

Backache is very common in pregnancy, affecting at least 50 per cent
of women, especially in the later stages. There are two main causes.
First, as your baby grows, the weight of your abdomen can pull the
lower spine forwards, so that it curves. This causes strain on lower back
muscles. Then your shoulders tend to pull back to compensate, and this
causes strain on the muscles in the upper back.

Pregnancy hormones soften and stretch ligaments, especially those
around the pelvis. This can make the joints in and around your pelvis
ache. Late in pregnancy, you may get backache if your baby settles in
your pelvis with its back lying against yours. Some women experience
backache as one of the first signs of the onset of labour.

Babyworld.co.uk members on backache:

▶ *Kepti says:* 'Try rolling a pillow up behind you while you sleep
to help support you. Keep yourself as straight as possible when sitting and standing up – with the extra weight up front it is easy to
find yourself slouching.'

▶ *Maya says:* 'I've found that keeping a hot water bottle on my
lower back for a couple of hours when I get home from work really helps me. I also sit on a birthing ball for at least 30-45 minutes a
day and I have got a very good chair at work.'

▶ *Luca says:* 'I try to get my husband to massage my back as
much as possible, but I often wake up in the night with pain around
my shoulder blades. I don't really like to wake him though, so then
I just resort to various stretches to try and ease my muscles.'

▶ *Gio says:* 'You could try sleeping with a pillow between your knees, or lying on your side. Also try doing a variety of slow stretches every few hours or so as that stops things getting so stiff and relaxes muscles.'

▶ *Pip 180 says:* 'Backache does tend to be more of a problem in later pregnancy, but it can occur in the early weeks too, due to the softening of muscles and ligaments. It might be worth asking your GP to refer you to a physiotherapist for advice on how to protect your back as pregnancy progresses.'

Top tips to ease backache

- Watch your posture. Rather than pushing out your abdomen, tilt your pelvis forward – as if you're pressing your lower back against a wall. Open out your shoulders and lift your rib cage.
- Careful lifting – when lifting heavy objects remember to squat and bend at the knees, never at the waist. Or just get someone else to do it.
- Ditch the stilettos – always wear, comfortable low heels.
- Support – put a cushion behind your lower back when you are sitting and sleep on a firm mattress.
- Talk to your midwife about getting a maternity girdle if the problem is severe.
- See an osteopath or chiropractor.
- If your backache is due to the position of your baby, kneel on all fours. This takes the weight of the baby off your back.
- Back pain can be caused by urinary infections. Try drinking cranberry juice or eating blueberries to ward off a UTI (urinary tract infection).

See also:

Pelvic pain – page 108

Babyworld.co.uk link: **www.babyworld.co.uk/faq**

> "I've had a couple of 'accidents' lately, leaking urine which is very embarrassing. Has this happened because I've not been doing my pelvic floor exercises?"

PELVIC FLOOR EXERCISES AND INCONTINENCE

Incontinence in pregnancy is not unusual, but it's not a common topic of conversation, so those who suffer usually do so in an embarrassed silence. This is a bit unfair, given that pregnancy incontinence is caused by a combination of 'stress', urinary infections and the relaxing effect of hormones on the pelvic floor. It's as much a part of the process for some women as nausea and tiredness, and it's important to acknowledge and address the issue.

'Stress incontinence' occurs at times when the internal pressure is raised – for example, when coughing, sneezing, lifting, vomiting or running. Although it is more common in the later stages of pregnancy, incontinence can affect women earlier, especially if they have had a baby already.

The best way to prevent incontinence is to practise pelvic floor exercises whenever you can. It is not advised to stop urinating mid-flow as a way of doing them, though, as this can cause urinary infections. The recommendation is that you do about 200 a day, a mixture of slow and fast twitches. It is important to continue your pelvic floor exercises after the birth as the risk of stress incontinence remains. Regular pelvic floor exercises will help tone the muscles for future pregnancies and may well help you avoid incontinence problems later in life.

Avoiding excessive weight gain and exercising regularly will also help reduce the risks of urinary problems. Though you will find that you will need to pass urine more frequently in pregnancy (due to hormonal changes), and you might find in the late stages of pregnancy that you occasionally leak a little urine, there is no reason to worry that you will become incontinent.

Babyworld.co.uk members on pelvic floor exercises:

▶ *KelD says:* 'These exercises aren't so much to help with the birth (although they do strengthen your muscles) it is more after, once everything has been stretched (birth canal etc.) it helps get things back to normal quicker'

▶ *TaraP says:* 'Even though you may not be doing lots of pelvic floor exercises, it is important to know where it is and how to do them. It is important to do post-natal exercises though. If you speak to women in their 60s, they will probably say that they wished they had done them. If you are unfortunate enough to do them but still have a problem you will know you did all you could.'

Babyworld.co.uk members on incontinence:

▶ *HollyG says:* 'I think it's possible to leak whether you have done 10 million pelvic floor exercises a day or not – it can just happen. It's reassuring to know that if or when I wet myself, I shouldn't panic as it's pretty normal.'

▶ *Gio says:* 'A bit of leakage may be down to the extra weight you're carrying on your bladder, and on your hormones. It is worth using pads so you have a back-up just in case. Keep practising the pelvic floor exercises, it may be worth doing them lying down so you don't have the weight of the baby on them.'

▶ *Mags01 says:* 'I have had a terrible cough for the past few days and I couldn't cough without wetting myself. Today I seem to have finally regained control of my bodily functions – for now anyway.'

See also:
Babyworld.co.uk link: **www.babyworld.co.uk/faq**

"I find myself going to the loo more often, and it's quite painful when I go – is there anything wrong?"

CYSTITIS

Midwife says: It's possible that you could be suffering from cystitis (a bladder infection). This is common in pregnancy, partly because of hormonal changes, which make the walls of the bladder softer, so it's harder to empty it, and partly because the growing uterus stretches your urethra, making it harder to pass water. If the bladder is not completely emptied, bacteria in the urine that's left behind can multiply and cause infection.

The good news is that cystitis, though painful and irritating, is not harmful to your baby. However, if a bladder infection is left untreated, it can lead to a kidney infection (pyelonephritis), which may be harmful to you and your baby, so if you have cystitis, you should take steps to treat it. It can sometimes be cleared by drinking lots of fluid to flush your bladder regularly, but if your symptoms persist for more than 24 hours, see your GP, as you may need antibiotics.

Babyworld.co.uk members on cystitis:

▶ *Suki says:* 'I have UTIs fairly often. Normally I drink loads of cranberry juice and it seems to go away on its own, though sometimes it gets progressively worse and I have to get antibiotics from my GP.'

▶ *Peta says:* 'Drink lots and lots of fluid. Barley water is good. Try to stay away from anything too acidic – I tend to dilute all fruit juice 50/50 with water as I find it a bit strong neat so that helps me down the requisite amount.'

▶ *Marthasmum says:* 'A colleague of mine who's a continence nurse gave me a tip which stopped my cystitis attacks and might stop you getting another infection. When you've finished you have to rock backwards and forwards a few times on the loo which swishes any urine that's left in your bladder around and stops it stagnating and causing an infection. You feel a complete idiot doing it but it has worked for me. You could also try laying off tea and coffee for a few days as they are both irritant to the bladder.'

▶ *Kat78 says:* 'One tip I did get at the hospital is that it is safe to take cranberry extract tablets which can help to keep things healthy. Good for me because I am not keen on the juice.'

Check your symptoms

Symptoms of **cystitis** include wanting to pass water more frequently – but only managing a few drops, a burning or stinging sensation when passing urine and a slight rise in temperature. It can lead to a 'heavy' feeling over your bladder and occasionally to traces of blood in your urine.

If you're feeling very unwell, with fever, pains in the abdomen, back or side and severe nausea or vomiting and your urine is dark or smelly contact your GP or maternity unit immediately, as these are possible symptoms of pyelonephritis.

See also:
Breast sensitivity and other early signs – page 10
Vaginal discharge – page 28
Babyworld.co.uk link: **www.babyworld.co.uk/faq**

"I find that I'm really gasping for breath walking home from work these days – am I just unfit or is there a more serious problem?"

SHORTNESS OF BREATH

When you're pregnant your lungs have to work much harder to meet your body's increased oxygen needs. To help you take in more air, your ribs flare out and your lung capacity increases dramatically. This can make you feel breathless, particularly from mid-pregnancy onwards.

In the last three months, most women find they get breathless even during mild exertion. This happens because your expanding uterus pushes up against the base of your lungs. Your breathing may start to get easier when your baby moves down into your pelvis ready to be born.

Women who are anaemic, or who are pregnant with more than one baby, may be particularly prone to breathlessness.

Babyworld.co.uk members on shortness of breath:

▶ *Bex10 says:* 'Strangely enough I suffered really badly from shortness of breath in the early stages of my pregnancy, long before baby was big enough to get anywhere near my lungs. I discovered that shortness of breath can be a sign of anaemia so I have been taking iron tablets ever since. I did have a blood test which indicated that I was anaemic and since then I have only had a few incidents of breathlessness which were due to baby squashing my lungs.'

▶ *Lilkat says:* 'My shortness of breath was apparently linked to SVT (a condition that creates an increased heart rate). Although it wasn't serious, it was still enough to cause me concern and make me stop and sit for a bit. Funnily enough when I was unable to walk and had to stay put, this stopped! Maybe the physical stress of caring for three kids, a baby and two dogs was too much for my poor old heart and lungs."

▶ *Mafi says:* 'I've started really struggling to breathe, like someone's sitting on me. Sometimes I just stand outside and get a few deep breaths of fresh air to bring me back to life. Other than that I have started to call on my family for more help.'

Take a breather with our tips

- Try to take things a bit slower and avoid rushing around – get some help with chores and shopping.

- Sleep propped up on several firm pillows if you get short of breath when you lie down.

- Practise deep breathing exercises, focusing on breathing out and letting your body relax. It's good practice for labour!

IMPORTANT: If you find you're feeling breathless even when resting, and/or it hurts to breathe, consult your doctor immediately.

See also:
Anaemia – page 36
Babyworld.co.uk link: **www.babyworld.co.uk/faq**

> **"I feel so sick all the time, it's really taking over my life. Surely this isn't normal pregnancy sickness?"**

SEVERE SICKNESS AND HYPEREMESIS

An extreme form of sickness in pregnancy is called hyperemesis. Women with hyperemesis find they need to vomit repeatedly (some up to 20 times a day) and the usual remedies make absolutely no difference. Hyperemesis can start at any stage of pregnancy but usually kicks in around four weeks and lasts until around 20 weeks. Sometimes it can last the entire pregnancy. Women with hyperemesis typically lose between five and 25 per cent of their weight in the first trimester.

While slight weight loss has no immediate detrimental effect on the baby, severe weight loss can cause foetal growth problems and can seriously affect the mother's health – in some severe cases it can even be life-threatening to the mother. Treatment for hyperemesis often involves hospitalization while medication is given to correct fluid balance.

Urinary tract infections may also cause nausea, vomiting and tiredness. A test taken by your midwife or GP should show whether there is an infection and whether it is sensitive to antibiotics. Antibiotics themselves may also make a woman feel unwell. If your symptoms are due to infection, they should settle once it is properly treated.

Babyworld.co.uk members on severe sickness and hyperemesis:

▶ *Peta says:* 'I've been finding the constant sickness so awful and as a consequence finding the experience of being pregnant very negative. It was the same with my first child. However, both times, at fourteen weeks, I have had reflexology. I find the sickness becomes so much more manageable, and I can feel more positive.

It really works for me – it could be good for you too. No harm in finding out.'

▶ *Tolmie says:* 'If I don't get something to eat within about two minutes of waking up I will be retching away for the next hour! Then I have to eat again about an hour later, and after that I'm OK. I find that if I'm tired it's much worse, so it's worth trying to get a few good nights' sleep if you have a bad patch.'

▶ *Nico8 says:* 'I think one of the hardest things about hyper-emesis is not knowing that you have it and wondering why you feel so unbelievably sick and other women don't. Once it is diagnosed that makes it easier to deal with. Some women have tried acupuncture, homeopathy and herbal remedies to help hypereme-sis. My personal experience is that acupuncture made it more bear-able. It never took my nausea away completely. I was able to func-tion and also able to eat small amounts.'

▶ *Sali says:* 'Unfortunately, around the end of the first trimester I started to feel violently sick every morning and was then physi-cally sick every single day until about 37 weeks when I stopped work. It was only first thing and pretty soon just became a sort of routine. Sometimes my toothbrush would set it off, sometimes get-ting up was enough. In the last few weeks of throwing up I could avoid actually vomiting by staying in bed until about 10am, but this was only possible at weekends. I think the stress of commut-ing and six months of trying to sort out my maternity leave arrange-ments was probably a contributory factor towards the end."

See also:
Morning sickness and nausea – page 20
Toothcare – page 50
Trying alternative remedies – page 136
Babyworld.co.uk link: **www.babyworld.co.uk/faq**

"I've read that there are recommendations for weight gain in pregnancy, but I'm nowhere near them – is something wrong?"

WEIGHT CHANGES

Midwife says: The opinion that women should gain weight in a specific way in pregnancy is actually no longer widely held. In fact, most midwives and doctors pay little attention to weight gain, as monitoring it has not been found to be of much benefit. A more individual approach is now usually taken, in which the woman's personal circumstances are considered more significant than statistics.

It is, of course, normal for women to gain weight during pregnancy, as a result of extra blood, extra fluid, bigger breasts, enlarged uterus, the placenta, amniotic fluid, the baby, as well as a store of fat as a reserve of energy for late pregnancy and beyond. However, the process of gaining weight can't be plotted on a straight line, nor can one woman's experience be compared directly with another's. Some women gain a lot of weight in the early weeks, while others only really begin to put it on in the later stages (and may even lose some at first). It's worth noting though, that rapid weight gain in later pregnancy, accompanied by sudden swelling, can be a sign of pre-eclampsia and should be checked out by your midwife or GP.

In general, if you're eating a balanced diet, including all the main food groups (but without lots of 'empty' calories), you aren't smoking, and you are managing to get some exercise (just 20 minutes brisk walking a day can help), then your weight gain is likely to be normal for you.

Babyworld.co.uk members on weight changes:

▶ *Mum2B says:* 'The key is to monitor what you are eating – if your diet hasn't increased dramatically in calories and weight is being gained then see your midwife or GP. It could be due to pre-eclampsia or other serious problems. The same goes for losing weight, though if weight is lost due to sickness then it is unlikely to harm the baby.'

▶ *Tez says:* 'Weight gain linked to pre-eclampsia is associated with fluid retention, so as long as you haven't suddenly swollen up as well, it's not likely to be anything to worry about.'

▶ *Suki says:* 'I lost 2kg right at the beginning of my pregnancy and have only put one back since. I think what's important is to ensure that we have a healthy and balanced diet."

▶ *Pip180 says:* 'I think it's normal that weight fluctuates (water retention or loss, eating a bit more or a bit less one day etc). So you might have lost a little compared to yesterday or a few days ago, but I think what's most important is that the general trend goes up. I know that in my case, I feel a lot more in touch with my body's needs and I feel like eating a lot more healthily than before I got pregnant, so that's why I'm not putting on much weight.'

▶ *Mili says:* 'Everybody's different, so don't take any notice of any charts telling you what you 'should' weigh. I know lots of women who lost weight in the first trimester due to constant vomiting and/or loss of appetite.'

▶ *Ami23 says:* 'I love being pregnant! I am really proud of my bump and who cares that I now weigh 13 stone. I'm eating sensibly and enjoying myself.'

See also:
Severe sickness and hyperemesis – page 72
Pre-eclampsia – page 106
Smoking, drinking and drugs – page 118
Keeping fit and exercising – page 120
Babyworld.co.uk link: **www.babyworld.co.uk/faq**

> **"I get sharp pins and needles in my hands and fingers.
> Sometimes it keeps me awake at night. What's wrong?"**

CARPAL TUNNEL SYNDROME

MIDWIFE SAYS:

It sounds like you might be suffering from carpal tunnel syndrome. This affects as many as one in three pregnant women, usually in the later stages when there is a lot of water retention.

The median nerve, which travels down your arm and into your hand, is crushed – either by inflammation, caused by repeated motion in the sleeve around it (the carpal tunnel) or by the pressure of water retention. This may lead to shoulder and elbow pain, pain in the centre of the wrist, and numbness or pins and needles in the thumb, index finger and middle finger. If you have pain in the little finger or ring finger you've got a problem with the ulnar nerve.

However, some women's experience of numbness and tingling in their arms and legs in later pregnancy is a result of their enlarging uterus pressing on a nerve. Moving into a different position to reduce the pressure sometimes helps. Pins and needles in your fingers may also be caused by the shoulder strap of your bra being too tight and pressing on the nerves that go into your arm.

Babyworld.co.uk members on carpal tunnel syndrome:

▶ *Peta says:* 'Don't be tempted to put on a compression bandage – that's the worst thing you can do. I found alternating heat and ice packs worked well for pain relief, and if you're working with a PC you must get the right equipment to give you a good typing posture. In the end, I had to switch hands and mouse with my left hand, using a giant mouse, a gel rest for the keyboard, and a very high-backed chair.'

▶ *Teri says:* 'I had carpal tunnel syndrome in my first pregnancy. Gradually it got worse and I was referred to a physiotherapist and was given splints to wear. They best helped me at night, as that was often the worst time, but as I work at a PC I also tended to wear the supports when I worked. I also found that at night I tried to make sure my hands were above my head as that helped too.'

▶ *Mum2B says:* 'It's a case of resting, ice packs and hanging your arm over the edge of the bed to get the blood flow going.'

▶ *SaraM says:* 'The best thing I find is to take off all your rings at night and if you get an attack of the tingles raise your hand in the air, this helps drain any excess fluid.'

Light at the end of the tunnel

- Other remedies that might help to ease the symptoms of carpal tunnel syndrome include:
- Try hand exercises – stretch your fingers out as far as possible then relax them. Repeat this a few times. Alternatively, make your hands into fists then stretch them out, or shake your hands around, using a 'flicking' motion.
- Use an improvised sling – a scarf or other soft material – to keep your hand elevated as often as possible.
- Consult a qualified acupuncture or acupressure practitioner.
- Ensure your diet includes vitamins from the B group, which keep your nerves healthy.
- Remember, not all remedies work for all women – if your symptoms are severe you may need to consult your GP for drugs to aid fluid loss.

See also:

Insomnia – page 78

Trying alternative remedies – page 136

Babyworld.co.uk link: **www.babyworld.co.uk/faq**

> **"I just don't sleep anymore – if I'm not uncomfortable, I can't stop worrying. How can I get some rest?"**

INSOMNIA AND SLEEPLESSNESS

Midwife says: Sometimes it can seem as if the symptoms of pregnancy are designed to keep you from sleeping. Pressure on your bladder, heartburn, restless legs and a fidgeting baby aren't exactly conducive to a good night's rest. But there are things you can do that might help you to get some rest.

If you're able to take naps during the day, that's obviously a good way to catch up on sleep, but otherwise when you go to bed, try and create the right environment for sleeping. Avoid caffeine from the afternoon onwards, and don't be tempted to eat a big meal late in the day. Try a night-time routine of doing some gentle exercise – a stroll round the block or some yoga stretches, perhaps – then a relaxing bath, a glass of water to keep you hydrated all night, and then straight to bed without reading or watching TV.

If you're being kept awake by worries about your baby or the birth, offload them by talking to your family or friends about them, or sharing them on babyworld.co.uk. Writing them down is another way of getting them off your mind. Once you've externalised your fears, it's often easier to rest and relax.

If you continue to find it impossible to sleep, though, speak to your GP. Also, if you find that you're sleeping well at night, but still feel tired in the daytime, this may be linked to factors such as anaemia, so it's important to get medical advice.

Babyworld.co.uk members on insomnia:

▶ *Han67 says:* 'My advice would be that if you haven't dropped asleep within 30 minutes then get up and do something productive

– like the ironing or the next day's lunches, which may then free up a bit of time the following day/evening so that if you feel tired you can nap then. I'd then try again after 30-60mins to see if I could get back off to sleep. Sometimes just getting up in a cold house then going back to bed 30 minutes later and snuggling down into a warm bed having had a milky drink was enough.'

▶ *Trixi says:* 'Trying to sleep in humid, hot conditions is awful. Investing in a couple of fans for your bedroom is the only way to go. My best advice though is to sleep where you are most comfortable. I have been on the sofa for several weeks now.'

▶ *Ozz says:* 'Last night I ended up getting up and rocking from side to side in an effort to quieten my moving baby. For the second time this week it worked! I've never thought to try it before but as they tend to wake up and fidget whilst you are resting, it makes sense to get up and rock them back to sleep.'

A little drop of something

No, we're not suggesting you down a nightcap (especially as alcohol dehydrates the body, meaning you're more likely to wake in the middle of the night). But if you've reached the last three months of your pregnancy, you might try putting some drops of lavender oil on your pillow (or in your bath) to aid sleep. Consult a qualified aromatherapist for more information on essential oils for pregnancy.

See also:

Tiredness – page 34

Anaemia – page 36

Smoking, drinking and drugs – page 118

Keeping fit and exercising – page 120

Relaxation techniques – page 138

Babyworld.co.uk link: **www.babyworld.co.uk/faq**

"**I've had such a miserable first trimester – when am I going to start blooming and feel better?**"

BLOOMING AND BOOSTED ENERGY

The fabled 'blooming' stage of pregnancy is a bit of an enigma. A wonderful shot in the arm for some, a bit of a disappointment for others and a total mystery for everyone else, it seems that blooming, like so much in pregnancy, cannot be predicted or relied upon.

Many women find themselves released from the draining early symptoms of pregnancy around 12-16 weeks and this can lead to an upsurge of energy as they find it easier to eat, sleep and work. Now isn't the time to overdo it – your body won't tolerate too much over exertion, but even if you don't think of yourself as a 'bloomer', you may be able to take advantage of increased energy levels to get some regular exercise, or even to take a holiday. The energy boost may not last forever – and it's worth making the most of it while you can.

A sizeable minority of women don't feel any better as the second trimester rolls on – with nausea, tiredness and other symptoms continuing unabated. Some may be distressed by other physical changes, such as weight gain or skin and hair changes. It's important to try taking the long view that almost all of pregnancy's downsides clear up as soon as the baby is born, but if you're feeling particularly down, or low on energy, it may be a sign of other problems, like anaemia. Speak to your midwife or GP for more advice.

Babyworld.co.uk members on blooming:

▶ *Kaylo says:* 'Glowing, blooming, I don't know what to call it but what I can say is that I haven't felt so good for a long time. Since the second trimester, I've been feeling good in my skin and very positive about life. I don't think it's anything in particular, more mood altering hormones for me and probably the excitement.'

▶ *TeriP says:* 'I would say that the blooming moments outweigh the non blooming. However I'm sure I felt different with my first pregnancy. I guess every day was exciting as I didn't know what to expect, whereas this time if I can't sleep or I have backache it is a pain rather than an exciting progression in my pregnancy.'

▶ *Gio says:* 'I like to think I'm blooming, but it depends on whether I've had enough sleep. I'm definitely looking and feeling better than 10 weeks ago, and I've been told I look really well by a few people. I've always had my suspicions though that 'well' means chubby. It is difficult to feel that you look OK when your waistline is disappearing before your eyes.'

▶ *Sami says:* 'People say I'm blooming, especially my husband, bless him – he keeps saying how gorgeous I look right now. I don't feel gorgeous however. My skin has greatly improved but I feel like a big heifer and not at all elegant!'

▶ *Lilkat says:* 'I don't think that the blooming stage exists for most of us, only for a very lucky few. I'm sorry to say that I was very spotty and greasy the whole way through last time, and it looks like I will be this time too. But I was back to normal within a couple of days of giving birth, so all the nastiness disappears very quickly afterwards.'

See also:
Anaemia – page 36
Your changing appearance – page 116
Keeping fit and exercising – page 120
Travelling while pregnant – page 144
Babyworld.co.uk link: **www.babyworld.co.uk/faq**

"I'm anxious to start feeling my baby's movements so I can feel more reassured that everything's fine. When do the movements start?"

FEELING THE BABY MOVE

If this is your first baby, you may feel the first 'fluttering' movements between 18-22 weeks. Women who have had a baby before may feel movement as early as 16 weeks, or sometimes even sooner – it's an unusual sensation and experienced mums have a better chance of distinguishing these movements from other body changes.

Some women find it hard to feel movements until much later on. If you have a very active lifestyle, you might miss these initial and very subtle sensations. Women who are larger than average may also find it more difficult to feel movements.

Once you've started feeling the baby's movements they can become a source of concern if they stop for any length of time. Again, it may just be that you've missed movements during a period of activity, but if you are in any way concerned about lack of movement contact your GP or midwife.

Babyworld.co.uk members on feeling the baby move (and waking it up):

▶ *HelenD says:* 'If you haven't started feeling movements it's possible that you're just too busy to notice, or it could be that the baby is in a position in which you can't feel anything, or the placenta is at the front of your uterus. This tends to cushion the movements so you can't feel them so easily.'

▶ *Mara says:* 'If your baby has been a bit quiet, eat something sweet. Ice cream, chocolate, orange juice – they all worked for me. Saves a trip to the hospital – although obviously if you are concerned, do go and get checked.'

▶ *Suse says:* 'Best advice I got was to lie still and close your eyes. You'll start to drift off to sleep and then the little worm goes and spoils it all by wriggling around.'

▶ *Peta says:* 'Remember that when you are out and about, you can't always feel anything anyway. The best time is always when it's quiet and you aren't rushing around as the movement tends to rock them to sleep.'

▶ *Marthasmum says:* 'If you are in any doubt or have worries call your midwife or hospital and ask their advice. I felt stupid for going in for some monitoring, as my baby dutifully kicked as soon as we got on the monitor, but they really didn't mind. I had spent a few hours worrying myself silly when I should have just got checked over earlier.'

▶ *AggieL says:* 'If you have a stubborn baby that refuses to move and is making life very uncomfortable for you with his elbow in your ribs or his feet on your bladder – eat something cold. It worked every time for me!'

See also:
Rib pain and stitches – page 60
Shortness of breath – page 70
Babyworld.co.uk link: **www.babyworld.co.uk/faq**

"This is my first pregnancy and I have no idea when my bump's supposed to start showing. What should I expect?"

BEGINNING TO SHOW

It's easy to see why many women – especially first-time mothers – want to see their bump. It is tangible evidence of pregnancy, letting the whole world in on the fantastic news. But there's no fixed rule for the development of a 'bump' – how soon you begin to show will depend on a range of factors including physical condition, height and weight.

First-time mums with taut stomach muscles may show later than mums with multiple pregnancies behind them. But that's not always the case. It's important not to worry about the emergence of your bump. If your midwife isn't concerned at your check-ups and scans haven't shown any problems, then your best bet is to relax and let nature take its course – if no one can see your bump at least they can't start grabbing it or worrying you about its size.

Babyworld.co.uk members on beginning to show:

▶ *Suki says:* 'With my first baby I was almost six months before you could tell. I actually had a pregnancy bump rather than a slightly bigger belly. Enjoy still being slim and don't stick your belly out as this will give you back ache.'

▶ *MelY says:* 'I didn't have a bump at 16 weeks, but I'm now 20 weeks and baby's presence is definitely known. Ignore what people say about the size of bumps, just say 'the baby's probably low down, and that's why you can't see my bump', that might stop them.'

▶ *Kara says:* 'Some people can be very insensitive – let them know that you really want a bump too and that they are making you worry unnecessarily. One of my friends was quite thin, and didn't start to show until really late – she was always aware that she was smaller than most people. One of her colleagues told her his wife was the same and at the end she was bigger than most people he'd seen. And that's exactly what happened to my friend. In the last two months she looked like she'd swallowed a beach ball – she looked fantastic.'

▶ *PamF says:* 'With my first pregnancy I was about five months before I looked remotely pregnant. I was desperate for a bump to appear! People are really rude – I was frequently told that I didn't look pregnant. My favourite was 'you don't look pregnant from behind!' No, I would say, that's because my uterus is at the front.'

▶ *Maya says:* 'I've got a bump this time, but then I've no stomach muscles left to speak of. If you started off with a flat, toned tummy then you'll hold the baby in more. Same if you are tall – there's more room for the baby lengthways, whereas if you're small, it can only come outwards. If you're slim, it'll take longer to show than if you've got a rounded tummy naturally. It all depends on your build.'

▶ *Teri P says:* 'Don't worry about what others say – and they always have a lot to say about bumps. As long as your midwife is happy with your size, that's all you need to worry about. All of a sudden it will arrive and you will then be moaning you have nothing to wear!'

▶ *Lorna23 says:* 'As soon as your bump appears it's as if you've got a neon sign above your navel saying 'feel free to feel me!' I've been quite taken aback by men diving in and touching this somewhat sensitive area without warning.'

See also:
Worrying about size of baby/bump – page 88
Your changing appearance – page 116
Maternity clothes – page 130
Babyworld.co.uk link: **www.babyworld.co.uk/faq**

> **"What are Braxton Hicks contractions? Will they hurt, and are they similar to 'real' contractions?"**

BRAXTON HICKS CONTRACTIONS

With a name like a firm of solicitors, Braxton Hicks sound formidable and worrying. But in fact these contractions are simply irregular tightening of the uterus. Although they happen from very early on, most women do not really notice them until the second half of pregnancy. Some may notice none at all throughout.

It is believed that these contractions help to tone the uterine muscle and promote the flow of blood to the placenta. Some people call them 'practice contractions'. They're usually started off by movement from you or the baby, or by someone touching your abdomen (for example during a check-up or scan).

Each 'contraction' may last a couple of minutes. During this time, the whole uterus becomes hard. This may feel strange and a bit uncomfortable – but shouldn't be painful. These contractions stay much the same throughout pregnancy, they do not get larger, harder or more frequent like 'real' contractions – though you may notice them more as time passes.

Braxton Hicks contractions are a normal and healthy part of pregnancy. If you're finding them uncomfortable, just try to relax and rest until they pass. If the contractions become more frequent or more painful over several hours or days – or if you lose blood or other fluid from your vagina – contact your GP or midwife straight away. This may be a sign of preterm labour.

Babyworld.co.uk members on Braxton Hicks contractions:

▶ *Kay67 says:* 'Some days I have bad Braxton Hicks. I normally feel them on a daily basis, and very easily if I do anything like climbing stairs, but on a couple of occasions I have had them with bad backache. As soon as they have gone, so has the back ache.'

▶ *LaraS says:* 'I have been feeling these for over a week now. The first three I felt were one a day over three days, and they were exciting. It felt weird – like your tummy tightens and it feels hard all the way into your ribs (but inside your body).'

▶ *Mia says:* 'I wasn't actually aware of any Braxton Hicks in my first pregnancy. It's so funny that some of us can feel them and others can't. Haven't felt anything this time yet either, and am wondering if this pregnancy will be the same'

▶ *Soren says:* 'It doesn't really matter if you notice them or not. Sometimes they are really obvious and can become quite regular and uncomfortable. In my last four pregnancies I spent three weeks before delivery having them every night and whenever I was walking!'

▶ *PhillyH says:* 'If you get a run of them move about. If you are sitting go for a walk, if you are moving, sit down. I find having a bath, taking a paracetamol, or quite often having a wee will make them either come or go!'

▶ *Katsmummy says:* 'Braxton Hicks should only be uncomfortable, never painful. If you have a warm bath and relax, see if they ease off. If they do, then you know you're not in labour. If they don't ease off, and you can see a pattern emerging then contact the hospital.'

See also:

Period-like cramps – page 16
Babyworld.co.uk link: **www.babyworld.co.uk/faq**

> **"I'm 28 weeks pregnant and my friend who is 18 weeks is huge next to me. Is there something wrong with my baby?"**

WORRYING ABOUT THE SIZE OF YOUR BABY/BUMP

Fears over a bump that is 'too large' or 'too small' are common in pregnancy, and particularly worrying in first pregnancies. It's easy to see why, as there's a lot of uninformed opinion bearing down on you from all sides. Unless your midwife or doctor has a specific concern, take comfort from the fact that many things can make a difference to the size of your bump at any given time – from clothing to posture to height, amount of body fat, amount of fluid around the baby, muscle tone, number of pregnancies and position of the baby.

Routine pregnancy scans will show up anomalies between the baby's size and your dates, while the most common medical condition that results in large babies is gestational diabetes and your midwife will be checking for this when she tests your urine. So take comfort from the fact that all women carry their babies slightly differently and that the size or prominence of bump is no indication of the size of baby. The most practical step you can take is to maintain a healthy, balanced lifestyle and let your body do its job.

Babyworld.co.uk members on worrying about the size of your baby/bump:

▶ *Yazi says:* 'The best thing to do if you're really worried is to chat to a midwife or consultant about a growth scan. Growth scans are not that reliable but it may help to reassure you. I think growth scans are probably a better idea if you're concerned that your baby is not growing well enough as they can measure the blood flow to the placenta and also along the umbilical cord. If this is not impeded then it's likely that baby is getting enough nutrients.'

▶ *Sal34 says:* 'I do think that the size of the bump and/or baby is one of the most anxiety-inducing problems during pregnancy, particularly for first-time mums. Everyone from consultants to mid-wives to passers-by seems to have some sort of comment about the size of the bump or the supposed size of the baby.'

▶ *LoriQ says:* 'I find the pressure to conform to a particular size is ridiculous. We all have different shaped bodies, and we should be looked at individually rather than conforming to the standard classification. All I can say is have confidence in yourself and your body, though when everyone else is busy sticking their nose in it can be so hard.'

Suki's story

'In my first pregnancy, I was 'small for dates' and didn't really have any bump to speak of for the first five to six months. By the final month, my midwife was making a fuss about my size. When I went overdue I declined induction, but was sent to a growth scan and told the baby was only 5-6lbs and was failing to thrive, so had to be induced. After a long and difficult labour, my 8lb 4oz baby was born!

'I think too much stress is placed on the size of the bump. A small bump doesn't necessarily equate to a small baby, just as a large bump won't necessarily lead to a large baby. The size of the baby is probably reliant on many other factors, such as maternal height and weight, genetics and nutrition.'

See also:
Gestational diabetes – page 100
Smoking, drinking and drugs – page 118
Babyworld.co.uk link: **www.babyworld.co.uk/faq**

"When I went to the loo this morning, I noticed some spots of blood. Am I going to miscarry?"

BLEEDING AND SPOTTING

Midwife says: Bleeding in pregnancy is always worrying, as it may be a sign of miscarriage. But bleeding is actually surprisingly common and in most cases when it happens, the pregnancy continues perfectly normally. If the bleeding is light and is not accompanied by cramps or sharp pain, the likelihood is that all will be well. Even a heavy bleed doesn't always mean that the pregnancy is miscarrying.

In early pregnancy, light bleeding or spotting can occur around the time that the woman would have been due her period. This happens because hormone levels aren't high enough to stop the bleeding, which comes from the lining of the uterus. Some women experience a light bleed following the implantation of the embryo – which is normally around 3-4 weeks, though the blood may come away later as a brownish discharge.

Spotting after sex is also fairly common throughout pregnancy, and as long as there's no pain associated with it, it is also nothing to worry about. Some women experience what's known as a 'cervical erosion' in pregnancy, which is a harmless change to the cells of the cervix that makes it prone to bleeding. Another cause of spotting may be urine or vaginal infections. It is always a good idea to mention any incidents of spotting to your midwife or GP.

Later in pregnancy, light bleeding can be a sign that labour is about to start, though a heavier, bright red bleed may be linked to problems with the placenta, which will require medical treatment. Again, let your midwife or GP know if you have any bleeding.

Babyworld.co.uk members on bleeding and spotting:

▶ *Maz says:* 'I had bleeding because of a low lying placenta, but it went away within a few days and I didn't have further problems.'

▶ *Pepi2 says:* 'In my first pregnancy I had light bleeding on and off from about six weeks to about 12 weeks. It was absolutely fine in the end and I now have a lovely healthy nine-month-old.'

▶ *Mum2B says:* 'I have been bleeding constantly since six weeks, with a very heavy bleed at about eight weeks and have had numerous scans and my baby is absolutely fine. I keep telling people this story as I was almost certain that things could not be OK, but I was proved very wrong.'

▶ *Teri says:* 'When I miscarried, the blood was persistent from five weeks onwards, and gradually picked up momentum. Light brown spots and streaks are most likely caused by an implantation bleed.'

▶ *Suze says:* 'Some women bleed throughout their pregnancy and as long as you are not having heavy bleeding or sharp, cramping pain in your stomach try not to worry.'

Bleeding – a checklist

- If you experience a bleed, it's always safer to let your midwife or GP know, but their advice will depend on the information you give about it. You should make note of the following:
- The colour of the blood (brown, dark or light red?)
- The quantity (a spot, a teaspoon, or enough to soak a sanitary pad?)
- Pain (any cramps, contractions or sharp jabs?)
- Frequency of baby's movements (in later pregnancy)
- The history of your pregnancy (including the results of ultrasounds and/or early scans)

See also:
Vaginal discharge – p28
Babyworld.co.uk link: **www.babyworld.co.uk/faq**

> **"I'm constantly worried that I'm going to miscarry. I just
> don't know how I'll cope if it happens to me."**

FEAR OF MISCARRIAGE

Midwife says: Easing the fear of miscarrying is a tough job, because
generally there isn't anything that can be done to prevent a miscarriage,
which can leave everyone feeling quite helpless in the face of this common trauma.

Statistics show that one in four pregnancies ends in miscarriage, but
this relates to all women, including those who are at a higher risk of miscarrying for some reason. It also includes very early miscarriages, which
are common and often occur before the woman is aware that she's
pregnant. It doesn't mean that every woman's risk of miscarriage is one
in four.

It's extremely common to worry about miscarrying in the early weeks of
pregnancy, and if you have any sustained cramping or heavy bleeds,
these should be reported to your midwife or GP, but even these symptoms don't necessarily mean that a miscarriage will follow. The risk of
miscarriage is highest in the first eight weeks, and by 12 weeks is small,
so hopefully by that stage you will be able to relax and enjoy your pregnancy.

There is no evidence to suggest that there's anything specific you can
do to avoid miscarriage, though maintaining a healthy lifestyle, eating a
well balanced diet and cutting down on alcohol and cigarettes helps
prepare your body for the demands of pregnancy.

Babyworld.co.uk members on fear of miscarriage:

▶ *Brumb says:* 'I think the fear of losing the baby is probably the
most overwhelming emotion during the first trimester for many
women. It can be quite anxiety-provoking to read statistics that

warn that as many as one in five pregnancies may end in miscarriage, and it does feel very strange having to tentatively say "IF the pregnancy goes OK, we could use this name/buy this/consider this...'

▶ *Teri says:* 'The 12/13 week mark is very significant. That knowledge that the risk has gone down and things are far more likely to succeed is very comforting, although I still think many women continue to worry about pregnancy loss until the birth.'

▶ *Marthasmum says:* 'I read that your chances of avoiding a miscarriage are improved by 15 per cent at six weeks and 95 per cent at eight weeks.'

▶ *Suse says:* 'In the end, we just have to relax. But the one thing I have decided to do is stop reading too much until my scan – it only worries me! If you try and take your mind off things, it does work!'

▶ *LaraP says:* 'I am pregnant again shortly after a miscarriage and know just how nerve-wracking this time is! When I was pregnant with my first child, I had very strong symptoms, yet had none at all when I miscarried. This time round, I didn't have many symptoms at all and naturally feared the worst. It was such a relief to have the 12 week scan and see that everything was OK!'

See also:
Period-like cramps – page 16
Feeling anxious – page 18
Bleeding and spotting – page 90
Miscarriage – page 94
Babyworld.co.uk link: **www.babyworld.co.uk/faq**

"I've miscarried. I feel so terrible, but no one seems to be able to tell me what went wrong or what I can do to make sure it never happens again."

MISCARRIAGE

Midwife says: A miscarriage is a terrible thing to experience, and the emotional impact can be huge. It's entirely understandable that you'd like to know why you miscarried, and how to prevent it from happening again, but actually most miscarriages occur because of random genetic abnormalities that mean the baby cannot develop properly. It is nature's way of ending a pregnancy that would not produce a baby, and is no one's fault. It's just chance.

Of course, it can be hard to rationalise the experience in this way and some women feel the need to seek the support of others who have been through the same experience, or to have counselling, to help them cope with their loss. Others feel that they want to start trying to conceive straight away, and miscarriages are often followed by successful, healthy pregnancies.

Although most miscarriages happen by chance, there are other possible, much less common, causes. These include abnormalities in the uterus or cervix, hormonal problems, factors like heavy smoking or drinking and drug abuse, infections such as rubella and toxoplasmosis, and severe or chronic illnesses like high fever, kidney disease, high blood pressure or blood clotting problems.

As a rule doctors don't investigate every miscarriage, but if a woman experiences three miscarriages in a row, tests are usually offered to explore possible causes for this. Having a miscarriage does slightly increase the chance of miscarrying in a subsequent pregnancy, but even after three miscarriages, the chances of the next pregnancy being successful is around 70 per cent.

Babyworld.co.uk members on miscarriage:

▶ *Maxi says:* 'When I miscarried, all I wanted was another baby, it became like an obsession. In hindsight, perhaps that wasn't the healthiest of reactions, but nevertheless our second son was conceived around three weeks after the miscarriage and the pregnancy was successful, though hugely stressful.'

▶ *Tula says:* 'Friends avoided us when we did miscarry, afraid they didn't know what to say or how to deal with it. That was as hurtful as the misguided comments some relatives made, such as "well it wasn't meant to be" and so on.'

Peta's story

'I felt unsettled during the weeks before I actually miscarried. Something felt 'wrong', to the extent that a tiny bit of spotting turned me into a nervous wreck despite the fact that I knew it was common in healthy pregnancies.

I wasn't surprised when my pregnancy miscarried, but I was surprised at the extent of my feelings. It's easy to see early pregnancy loss as 'one of those things', but when it happens to you it really does have a huge impact. I didn't realise I would feel so empty or cry so much.

I think after miscarriage, no pregnancy is ever the same again. You don't take it for granted that the baby will be fine, and I found we were more cautious about announcing the news to friends.'

See also:
Bleeding and spotting – page 90
Fear of miscarriage – page 92
Telling your family – page 112
Babyworld.co.uk link: **www.babyworld.co.uk/faq**

"I'm getting pain in my abdomen and I've heard this can be a sign of ectopic pregnancy. What should I do?"

ECTOPIC PREGNANCY

Midwife says: An ectopic pregnancy occurs when the embryo becomes embedded outside of the uterus. In almost all cases this will happen in one of the fallopian tubes linking the ovaries to the uterus. As the embryo develops, the tube is unable to stretch with it, leading to chronic pain, bleeding and ultimately, if not detected in time, a burst tube, which can pose a serious risk to the mother's health.

An ectopic pregnancy is a serious condition, but it is sometimes hard to diagnose in the early stages. This is because the initial symptoms of an ectopic pregnancy are the same as those of a normal pregnancy – missed periods, tender breasts, nausea etc. Symptoms that suggest that a pregnancy could be ectopic include, particularly between four and ten weeks, a constant, chronic one-sided pain in the lower abdomen, dark brown watery bleeding, dizziness, a racing pulse, pain when passing urine or opening your bowels, heavy vaginal bleeding or pain in the shoulder. If you experience any of these symptoms you should consult your GP immediately.

Treatment for an ectopic pregnancy is normally its removal under general anaesthetic. The affected tube may also need to be removed. Sometimes, particularly if the condition is discovered early on, it's possible for it to be treated by an injection to destroy the cells. The reasons behind an ectopic pregnancy are often hard to establish – though possible causes include the fallopian tubes being scarred due to previous infections or surgery, the use of a contraceptive coil and chlamydia.

Suffering an ectopic pregnancy doesn't necessarily make you more prone to another one in the future, but you may well be offered more scans to check the progress of subsequent pregnancies if you are deemed to be at risk.

Babyworld.co.uk members on ectopic pregnancy:

▶ *Suki3 says:* 'When I had the ectopic the pain was chronic – I couldn't stand up straight – and I was also bleeding.'

▶ *NewKaren says:* 'Shoulder tip pain can be a sign of ectopic pregnancy. Apparently the shoulder pain will be really quite strong if associated with an ectopic – bleeding from the ectopic presses on the nerves in your diaphragm, which link to your shoulder.'

▶ *Mum2B says:* 'Pain from an ectopic is persistent and severe. Other symptoms of an ectopic are dark brown watery bleeding (like prune juice).'

▶ *Gio says:* 'I've had not one but two early scans! This is because I had an ectopic pregnancy five months after my first son was born and lost a tube. There can be an increased risk of another ectopic if you've already had one, so I was told to have early scans after that.'

See also:
Fluctuating symptoms – page 14
Period-like cramps – page 16
Bleeding and spotting – page 90
Babyworld.co.uk link: **www.babyworld.co.uk/faq**

"I'm feeling really run down, but I'm petrified of getting ill in case I pass something on to my baby. What are the risks?"

GETTING ILL

Midwife says: The two main areas of concern regarding illness in pregnancy are avoiding infections that can be passed on to your baby, and ensuring you use the correct treatments when dealing with common illness (coughs and colds etc).

Let's deal with the infections first. Most infections, including coughs and colds, don't actually pose any risk to the baby, but there are some that do, particularly in the early weeks. These include rubella, chickenpox and cytomegalovirus (CMV), which can lead to birth defects, and measles, mumps and slapped cheek disease, which carry an increased risk of miscarriage. If you've come into contact with any of these viruses and aren't sure whether you're immune to them, consult your GP for a blood test.

As regards treatment for minor illnesses, it's always best to avoid medication in pregnancy where possible, though it's regarded as being OK to take paracetamol, in the standard dose, for pain relief or to ease the symptoms of a cold, if you want to. It's best not to take any other types of medication without consulting your GP or a pharmacist.'

Babyworld.co.uk members on getting ill:

▶ *D1974 says:* 'My son had chicken pox when I was about three weeks pregnant and didn't know it. I had it when I was seven, but wanted to make sure that I had retained my immunity. Fortunately I had, but if they find out that you haven't then they can give you an injection to give you some immunity so you and baby will be OK, but they need to do this early on.'

▶ *Petal says:* 'If a woman catches chickenpox in the first 20 weeks of pregnancy, there is a small risk (1-2 per cent) of the baby being affected, but this means that 98-99 per cent of babies whose mums have chickenpox in the first half of pregnancy are fine, although after 36 weeks the risk to the baby from a maternal infection can be as high as 50 per cent.'

▶ *TreyP says:* 'See your GP. Remember that most medicines are in fact safe in pregnancy but manufacturers don't want to be sued and so if you have to take something that isn't advised it is very unlikely to cause harm. Often taking something can reduce the risks of your illness harming the baby so is a good idea anyway.'

▶ *Mum2B says:* 'For coughs, colds and sore throats I've always used a hot honey, lemon juice drink to sooth away the aches and pains, along with some Paracetamol. I find it tastes much nicer than the sachets of cold and flu remedies and does pretty much the same job.

I am trained in massage too, and find that a facial drainage massage works wonders on blocked sinuses – and reflexology is fantastic too.'

See also:
Cravings – page 22
Pets and babies – page 128
Trying alternative remedies – page 136
Babyworld.co.uk link: **www.babyworld.co.uk/faq**

"I've been told I've got gestational diabetes. Does this mean I'll have to inject insulin – and will it harm my baby?"

GESTATIONAL DIABETES

Midwife says: A diagnosis of gestational diabetes is made when a pregnant woman has raised blood sugar levels because her body's insulin isn't working as it should. You may be more likely to develop gestational diabetes if there's a family history of diabetes, or if you're an older mother or are overweight.

Gestational diabetes may be suspected if you have high levels of sugar in your urine or if there's a lot of fluid around your baby or the baby is big. It's screened for by doing a glucose tolerance test (GTT). The main effects of gestational diabetes on the baby are that he or she may grow large, which can complicate labour, and may develop low blood sugar after birth. Both of these are less likely to happen if the diabetes is well controlled. Usually, it's possible to control it through regular self-monitoring of blood sugar levels and modifying your diet – you'll be referred to a diabetic clinic for advice on this – although in a small number of women, insulin needs to be given.

Women who have gestational diabetes will not become diabetic after the pregnancy, but they do run an increased risk of developing the condition again in future pregnancies. If it's correctly monitored and managed, the risks to the baby are small and it's usually possible to have a normal birth.

Babyworld.co.uk members on gestational diabetes:

▶ **Pepi says:** 'I've had glucose traces in my urine samples at every midwife appointment and had a glucose tolerance test. I come in a high risk category being over 35 and both my parents were diabetic. Luckily mine was negative, but even if positive it doesn't necessarily mean you will have to take insulin.'

▶ *Tessa71 says:* 'I've got gestational diabetes and have to test my blood four times a day with a machine the hospital provided. As for the diet, it's basically cutting out sugar and fat. I use a sweetener, and get my 'sweet' cravings fixed with sugar-free jelly with low fat fromage frais mixed in! I just think of it as a head start on the dieting after baby is born!'

▶ *Marthasmum says:* 'The worry is that babies born to diabetics tend to be large for dates and suffer after birth due to abnormal blood sugar levels. If sugar levels can be kept as normal as possible there is less risk of this happening.'

▶ *Kaza says:* 'Some doctors may recommend early induction out of a genuine concern for mother and baby but since scans are not good for predicting size some babies are born small and premature. I have seen this happen and it's worrying.'

Pip180's story

'I developed gestational diabetes in my last pregnancy, so this time round I'm trying to reduce my chances of getting it again. I'm much more aware of foods and nutrition and the effect they have on the body. I'm making sure I eat slow-releasing carbohydrates. I'll have either porridge or muesli on waking, then at about 10.30am I have a snack of carrots or a banana (good for fibre). I keep lunch really simple – organic soup and a slice of wholemeal bread (more fibre). At around 3pm another snack of crackers or fruit and then dinner around 5pm – tonight was lasagne.'

See also:

Worrying about the size of baby/bump – page 88
Keeping fit and exercising – page 120
Babyworld.co.uk link: **www.babyworld.co.uk/faq**

"My friend was a carrier of Group B Strep, and had antibiotics in labour – why haven't I been tested for it in my pregnancy?"

GROUP B STREP

Midwife says: Group B Streptococcus (GBS) is a bacteria carried in the gut of around one third of adults. It can also be carried, on an on and off basis, in the vagina. It is mostly harmless to the carrier, though it can lead to vaginal or urinary infections.

However, it does pose a small risk to an unborn baby, particularly if the mother has it in her vagina at the time of the birth, when it can be passed on to the baby. Fewer than half of the mothers who carry GBS will pass it on to their baby during birth and of those babies who do pick it up, just one per cent will become ill. But the illnesses caused by GBS can be serious ones, like meningitis, pneumonia and septicaemia, so once a mother is found to carry the bacteria, treatment with antibiotics during labour is recommended, to prevent it from being passed to the baby.

GBS isn't routinely tested for during pregnancy because the test that's available on the NHS is not very reliable, and fails to detect a high proportion of cases. It is, however, possible to have a test done privately, which offers greater reliability. If you are found to carry GBS, don't worry – having antibiotics during labour will protect the baby. If it's not known whether you carry it or not, you may still be offered antibiotics if your labour is premature (before 37 weeks) or your waters break prematurely (before 37 weeks), if you have a raised temperature in labour, or if your waters have been broken for longer than 24 hours, as these are circumstances in which, if you were to be a carrier, the likelihood of the baby picking the bacteria up is increased.

Babyworld.co.uk members on Group B Strep:

▶ *Gio says:* 'Some hospitals don't automatically induce you if you have GBS, but if there is any suggestion of your waters breaking and no sign of labour within a certain time then they may induce you. Make sure you let them know if you are allergic to penicillin as that may be one of the antibiotics used.'

▶ *Pip180 says:* 'My friend had GBS with her first pregnancy but she didn't know until she was in her second! The second time round she was told to get into hospital when the contractions were five minutes apart so they would have enough time to get the antibiotics through her system to avoid the baby having to have them!'

▶ *Kaza says:* 'I have no problem that the NHS don't offer a test. But it bothers me that no one seems to know about it or about testing. My midwife kept all the info I had to read up on it! Had I not known someone who suffered a loss due to this, I would have never known it existed.'

▶ *Tempo5 says:* 'I had to have intravenous antibiotics every four hours during labour (in my case during induction) to allow time for the antibiotics to pass through the placenta to the baby before delivery. If you want to know more about Group B Strep, visit www.gbss.org.uk – this is the UK charity and support group.'

See also:
Antenatal appointments – page 146
Babyworld.co.uk link: **www.babyworld.co.uk/faq**

"My bloods have come back and I'm rhesus negative. What does this mean and will it harm my baby?"

RHESUS NEG AND ANTI-D

Midwife says: Most people's red blood cells are rhesus positive, but in around 15 per cent of people, they're rhesus negative. Your rhesus status is significant in pregnancy because if you're rhesus negative and your partner is rhesus positive, your baby may also be rhesus positive. This is an issue because if any of a rhesus positive baby's blood cells get into a rhesus negative mother's bloodstream – which can happen, for example, if the mother has a bleed, or a heavy fall, or a procedure such as amniocentesis – then the mother's body will produce antibodies which can attack the baby's red blood cells.

Low levels of antibodies aren't usually harmful to the baby, but high levels can cause serious problems for him/her. The risk of antibodies developing can be countered by giving the mother an injection of a substance called anti-D, which prevents antibodies from forming. In a lot of areas, anti-D is offered routinely to all pregnant women who are rhesus negative at around 28 and 34 weeks. Once a dose has been given, it is effective for up to six weeks. Anti-D is given after birth as well (usually following blood tests on mother and baby), as the baby's blood can come into contact with the mother's during birth.

Anti-D is also given to any rhesus negative women who experience bleeding after 12 weeks of pregnancy – before 12 weeks there is only a very small risk of your baby's blood entering your bloodstream – or following other events as a result of which the baby's blood could come into contact with yours. The process of testing for antibodies and giving anti-D will be repeated for each pregnancy you have.

Babyworld.co.uk members on Rhesus negative and anti-D:

▶ *Sooz says:* 'I am Rhesus negative and have three healthy little boys so don't panic. With my first I had lots of little bleeds throughout the pregnancy and they gave me anti-D each time.'

▶ *Bell20 says:* 'They are so much better at testing these days – in the past (our mum's generation) they couldn't tell if there was a problem until the baby was born, but now they can pick problems up very early and deal with them.'

▶ *FranP says:* 'Warning, if they do give you the injection – it hurts! They have to inject it into your muscle rather than a vein, and you can feel the stuff going in. But in my opinion a few seconds of pain is worth it for not having to worry about my Rhesus status.'

▶ *Jaz says:* 'The injections are uncomfortable! I always have it in the top of the thigh or buttock area as it doesn't seem to ache as much.'

See also:
Bleeding and spotting – page 90
Babyworld.co.uk link: **www.babyworld.co.uk/faq**

"I've been getting abdominal pain and I'm really worried it might be the first sign of pre-eclampsia. What are the other symptoms?"

PRE-ECLAMPSIA

MIDWIFE SAYS:

Pre-eclampsia is a potentially dangerous pregnancy complication, which poses risks to both mother and baby. The main problem with diagnosing it is that the individual symptoms of pre-eclampsia are common in pregnancy and are usually harmless in isolation. However, the 'classic' signs of pre-eclampsia are high blood pressure, protein in the urine, and swelling of the face, hands, legs and feet, and when these occur together, this generally points to pre-eclampsia, which will require medical treatment.

Other symptoms that can be associated with pre-eclampsia include severe headaches, disturbed vision, nausea and/or vomiting and upper abdominal pain. Any of these symptoms should be reported to your midwife or GP.

When pre-eclampsia is diagnosed, it's usually managed by regular monitoring (blood pressure checks, urine tests and blood tests) and sometimes by blood pressure medication. Rest is advisable.

While in its early stages, the mother generally feels quite well, in its advanced stages, pre-eclampsia can affect her circulation, liver, kidneys, heart and central nervous system, and if the point is reached where the risks to the mother's health outweigh the benefits to the baby of remaining in the uterus, or there are signs that the baby is being affected (such as their growth being restricted), a decision is taken for the baby to be born early.

Babyworld.co.uk members on pre-eclampsia:

▶ *Tizz says:* 'Pre-eclampsia symptoms can include swelling of the hands and face, headaches, and stomach pain in your upper bump as well as raised blood pressure and protein in your sample. Flashing lights can also be a sign of pre-eclampsia – if you're suffering any of these you ought to get them checked by your GP.'

▶ *Han67 says:* 'If you're getting abdominal pain, have a gentle feel of your ribs – if it is worse when you press them it is likely to be ligament pain, if it doesn't make a difference it could be the baby moving and pushing up against your ribs or it could be a sign of pre-eclampsia.'

▶ *Peto says:* 'If you do have pre-eclampsia, it may become necessary for the baby to be born early, although they will always be left where they are for as long as possible. It isn't always the case that a caesarean is needed, though. Inducing labour is an alternative.'

See also:
Headaches – page 26
Swollen ankles, legs and fingers – page 32
Shortness of breath – page 70
Weight changes – page 74
Babyworld.co.uk link: **www.babyworld.co.uk/faq**

"I'm suffering from increasingly bad pelvic pain. What could be causing it?"

PELVIC PAIN

MIDWIFE SAYS: Mild pelvic discomfort is a common symptom in pregnancy as your ligaments loosen to prepare the pelvis for birth. However, more extreme discomfort, ranging through to chronic pain, is a sign that there's a dysfunction in the pelvic area which may require treatment and support as the pregnancy advances.

The most common form of pelvic dysfunction is symphysis pubis dysfunction (SPD) which is caused by the pubic joint not working as it should. This causes pain in the pubic area, groin, inside thighs and sometimes the lower back and hips.

It's advisable for women who have SPD to be seen by an obstetric physiotherapist, who can recommend ways of modifying their lifestyle to minimise the impact on the affected areas. Women with SPD are also often supplied with a special support belt to wear. Painkillers might also be needed. In extreme cases, crutches, or even a wheelchair, need to be used.

The most severe form of pelvic pain is diastasis symphysis pubis (DSP), which involves the pubic joint separating by more than 1cm. This isn't common (it affects 1 in every 500-800 women) but is very painful and debilitating. SPD usually gets better within a few months of the baby being born.

Babyworld.co.uk members on pelvic pain:

▶ *Mum2B says:* 'If you have SPD, then try and keep your knees as close together as possible. Take small steps when you walk, go up and downstairs like a toddler, sit down to get dressed, and when you get in and out of bed (or a bath or the car), sit with your knees together and swing your legs round.'

▶ *SukiX says:* 'The only thing I've found that helps is resting up for a few days. My midwife is fabulous and she's put me in touch with another local midwife who practises Reiki and Reflexology for SPD.'

▶ *Gio says:* 'My midwife was brilliant, and immediately referred me to an obstetric physiotherapist who gave me loads of advice, a brace to wear, crutches and telephone support as I needed it. I found that I had to ask for the referral though, and didn't just get it, although once I had asked it was quite smooth from there.'

▶ *D1974 says:* 'If it's not actually SPD that you have then it's simply a case of adapting your routine for now and pacing yourself. I've found this time that picking up my 1-year-old was aggravating the pain enormously – since he's been walking it's been much better.'

▶ *Pip180 says:* 'I am suffering with SPD too, I wear something silky to bed if possible, as it makes turning over easier. Swimming helps too, but avoid the breast stroke.'

Pelvic Pain – some myths

If you suffer from DSP or SPD you can't deliver your baby naturally – FALSE. Neither complaint stops a natural delivery, but the midwives and medical staff attending your delivery should be fully briefed about the condition so they make every effort to avoid worsening it.

DSP only occurs during pregnancy – FALSE. While most women experience a gentle lessening of the pain from DSP after giving birth, some only start to experience the condition post-delivery.

See also:

Babyworld.co.uk link: **www.babyworld.co.uk/faq**

> **"I can't stop itching – is this normal in pregnancy, or is there something wrong with me?"**

ITCHING AND OBSTETRIC CHOLESTASIS

Midwife says: Itching is a common irritation at various stages of pregnancy. Generally, it is linked to the stretching of your skin (over your bump, or breasts, for example) or to hormonal changes. Itching in the first few weeks of pregnancy is most likely to be either hormonal or perhaps some kind of allergic reaction.

There are various rashes that can develop in pregnancy, which can also cause itching. One of the most common is PUPP (pruritic urticarial papules and plaques of pregnancy), also known as toxic erythema, which sounds rather alarming, but is actually like a type of nettle rash. This commonly starts on the belly. The only way to identify what any particular rash is, and to ensure the right course of treatment, is to get it checked by your GP.

Itching can also be a symptom of a pregnancy-related liver condition called obstetric cholestasis, which can be harmful for mother and baby, so all itching should be reported to your GP or midwife as a precaution. Obstetric cholestasis doesn't usually develop till the last three months of pregnancy, it has no associated rash and the itching isn't limited to your belly. An early diagnosis, close monitoring and the use of drugs can help to manage the condition and limit risk – though because there's a risk to the baby if the pregnancy continues past 37-38 weeks, it's usual for steps to be taken for the baby to be born around this time. The condition normally clears up soon after the birth.

Babyworld.co.uk members on itching:

▶ *Pip180 says:* 'I was prescribed Hydrocortisone cream for my itching, which I have tried not to use too much, but am now putting it on twice a day. The other thing that I find really helps is putting cold wet flannels on the itchy area – especially when I'm having a scratching episode in the middle of the night!'

▶ *Trixi says:* 'Try aqueous cream with calamine, keep it in the fridge so it's nice and cool when applied. If you dab cool water with bicarbonate of soda in it onto your itchy areas it may help. I was told that Piriton antihistamines are safe to take, but consult your GP first.'

▶ *D1974 says:* 'Another thing you could try is having an oatmeal bath. Put a handful of oatmeal in a hanky or some old tights, tie it round the taps and let the water run through it. Don't have your bath or shower water too hot as that can make itching worse.'

▶ *Teri says:* 'I have a rash on my bump. It started on the underside of my bump and then went to the top and then the sides. The rash was very small bumps which itched like mad. The doctor said that it was just one of those things and to try to moisturise it as much as possible – they have now gone though my belly is still itchy but instead of scratching it I now moisturise.'

▶ *Marthasmum says:* 'I find that covering my legs with cotton pyjamas and standing outside in bare feet in the cold helps.'

See also:
Babyworld.co.uk link: **www.babyworld.co.uk/faq**

"When is the best time to tell my family and friends our good news – should I wait until 12 weeks?"

TELLING FAMILY AND FRIENDS

There's no right answer to this one – it really is a matter of personal choice and individual circumstance.

The main factor that stands in the way of shouting your good news from the rooftops is the possibility that the pregnancy may end in a miscarriage. As we've seen, the risk of this decreases sharply by 12 weeks, which is why some couples choose to hold back the news until they feel certain that all will be well. If you tell no one, then you won't have to break the sad news either – but you'll also go without their support or understanding. It's a difficult balancing act and one that you should consider carefully before excitement and enthusiasm take over.

Of course, some women don't have the luxury of waiting, especially if their symptoms are pronounced from the offset, while others find that waiting a little longer to share the news allows them and their partner more time to adapt to the idea of impending parenthood without constant 'advice' from friends and relatives.

Babyworld.co.uk members on telling family and friends:

▶ *Sali says:* 'I couldn't keep it a secret for very long. I initially felt really awkward about telling anyone, including my mum, because even at 29 I don't really feel like a grown up sometimes! However, once we started telling people it was nice because they were really happy for us, and it gave me a nice warm fuzzy feeling realising how much people care. Although my mother's comment was "it's about time".'

▶ *Marthasmum says:* 'I was so sick we told our families when I was only about 7 weeks. At the time I felt so ill, that was all I could think about – but so many people were really excited for us, it was lovely!'

▶ *Rady says:* I've not told very many people at all. My last pregnancy ended in miscarriage and I just feel that I want to be sure that everything is OK with this one before I announce it to all and sundry.'

▶ *Megs says:* 'Lots of people leave it until they've had their scans or test results. People will understand if you tell them that you just wanted to be sure that everything was OK.'

▶ *Loli67 says:* 'At the end of the day, you can only tell people when you feel comfortable and happy to do so. With my son, we told everyone within a couple of days of finding out. However this time around we have only told close family and a couple of friends. I can't wait to tell everyone but think I'll hold off until after my 12 week scan.'

▶ *Lilkat says:* 'I've told anyone who is interested. The way I look at it is I'm very much a heart on my sleeve person, and if I lose this baby then everyone will see me wailing so they may as well know the reasons before hand. It's no crime to lose a baby and I'll need support from the people around me.'

▶ *MiaJ says:* 'There is no right and wrong at all – just depends on how you feel you would cope if things went wrong – would you want people to know? If you feel 'yes, you want as much support as possible' then you have done the right thing. I'm a 'bury my head in the sand' kind of person so I would like to keep it to myself should things go wrong.'

See also:
Telling your work – page 114
Babyworld.co.uk link: **www.babyworld.co.uk/faq**

> "When is the best time is to tell people at work? I want everyone to know I'm pregnant, but I'm not keen on being treated differently."

TELLING YOUR WORK

You don't need to tell your employer that you're pregnant until 15 weeks before your estimated week of delivery. However, if you work in a job that may put you or your baby at risk, you should tell your employer immediately.

Many women wait until they have had their first scan at around 12 weeks before announcing their pregnancy, but if you're suffering from sickness, tiredness or other early symptoms that require you to take time off work, letting your employer know about the pregnancy ensures your absence is logged as pregnancy-related. Pregnant women are allowed 'reasonable' amounts of paid leave to attend antenatal appointments. Your employer may ask for written confirmation that you are pregnant and proof of your appointments. You can get an appointment card from your midwife or GP at your first antenatal appointment.

Another advantage of announcing your pregnancy is that you may be able to adjust your workload, especially if your job involves standing, lifting, or carrying. All pregnant women are entitled to health and safety protection at work to ensure that working conditions do not put them, or their baby, at risk. If you are concerned about your working conditions, ask for a risk assessment. To find out more, contact your union representative, HR department or your local Health and Safety Executive.

It is against the law for your employer to sack you or make you redundant for any reason connected with pregnancy, childbirth or maternity leave. This applies from day one of your pregnancy. You are protected no matter how long you have worked for your employer. If you are being treated unfairly, seek advice from your union or local Citizens Advice Bureau.

Babyworld.co.uk members on telling your work:

▶ *Olmo says:* 'It is a good idea if your work knows earlier rather than later for health and safety reasons – once I knew I was pregnant I refused to carry boxes of stationary or lug postbags around.'

▶ *Hari says:* 'Don't expect others to share your joy. Sometimes people see your pregnancy as an inconvenience or a hassle, they might have to do more work to cover you and they don't always like it. But know your rights, they cannot sack you for being pregnant, you are entitled to take antenatal care appointments, and you can ask for a risk assessment to be carried out if you think your job may harm you or the baby. This goes for women who work nights as well, and you also have many rights if you are a part time employee.'

▶ *Suse says:* 'You are only legally obliged to tell your boss by the 25th week of pregnancy, but if you want time off before then, even for a medical appointment, a caring and understanding boss should be OK. If I find myself pregnant again I think I would wait until I was 10 weeks or so to avoid it being a 'long' pregnancy at work.'

▶ *Mags01 says:* 'I've worked at the same company since before my first pregnancy. With my first I told work when I was 11 weeks, with my second I was 13 weeks. Both times they were brilliant and let me have any time off I needed for appointments, and if the appointment was late afternoon, I wasn't expected to go back to work afterwards.'

▶ *Trixi5 says:* 'Last time I was pregnant I told HR as soon as I found out in case I got sick or had a miscarriage. Then I told my boss at 12 weeks, followed by a big announcement to my team.'

See also:
Maternity leave – page 140
Babyworld.co.uk link: **www.babyworld.co.uk/faq**

"I've always been very proud of my figure and it's a bit hard to face the idea that I'm just going to get big in pregnancy. Will I lose all my self-confidence?"

YOUR CHANGING APPEARANCE

We've already discussed the changes that are happening to your body in cold detail (stretch marks, beginning to show, swollen ankles) and each of these can be analysed in turn. What we struggle to do is assess the whole experience, as first one part of your body then another becomes alien to you.

For some women this is the worst part of pregnancy – they feel invaded. For others it's like growing a new skin. They feel invulnerable, confident and special. Where you sit between the two camps depends on many factors, including your self-confidence before pregnancy, the supportiveness of your partner, family and friends and your general health in pregnancy to date.

There is no 'right' attitude in pregnancy, whatever other people may say. Whether you view pregnancy as something to be endured or embraced, it's worth maintaining a positive outlook and a healthy lifestyle. This will help you enjoy the highs and cope with the lows. Most of the symptoms you're experiencing will clear up after the birth, but if you need reassurance over your changing appearance, speak to your midwife.

Babyworld.co.uk members on their changing appearance:

▶ *MayaL says:* 'I love my children to bits and I wouldn't change them at all, but I HATE being pregnant. I hate the way my body changes and how I grow outwards. I really can't stand getting larger and larger, even though I know I am having a baby. I used to hate wearing maternity clothes because they never fitted properly, and I used to find that I was so uncomfortable in the evenings I used to sit around in maternity nightwear. I would love a third child but can't face getting large in pregnancy again.'

▶ *Lilkat says:* 'I adore being pregnant. I suffer quite badly with self esteem issues but they go out of the window in pregnancy and I love having that confidence.'

▶ *LoriQ says:* 'Once my bump finally appeared properly I loved the ripe pregnant look. Before that it was a bit miserable as I just looked fattish. I actually lost weight in the first trimester which was not ideal. I had no stretch marks at all until 36 weeks when I got up one morning and the underside of my bump was covered in vile purple marks.'

▶ *Usper says:* 'For me, the most upsetting parts of my appearance during pregnancy were that my ankles were hugely swollen like an old lady's, my eczema, which was already bad, got a lot worse and then I got stretch marks. My husband says these are fabulous. He is fascinated by them. Not sure if he's just being nice, but they certainly don't seem to put him off!'

▶ *TeriP says:* 'I was so happy to be pregnant and enjoyed the whole experience – although admittedly I did have it really easy, but I think the way partners' feel about your changing figure has more effect than they may think.'

▶ *Lottie6 says:* 'Once you could tell I was pregnant I loved my shape. I loved sticking my bump out proudly and feeling the baby kicking. I was forever rubbing my belly.'

See also:
Stretch marks – page 56
Swollen ankles – page 62
Beginning to show – page 84
Partner's attitude – page 126
Maternity clothes – page 130
Babyworld.co.uk link: **www.babyworld.co.uk/faq**

> "I'm trying to quit smoking and drinking, because I don't want to harm my baby – but it's SO hard. Please help"

SMOKING, DRINKING AND DRUGS

Midwife says: First of all, well done for taking the step of trying to stop smoking and drinking. That takes a lot of courage and deserves support. Of course, the best way of ensuring that your baby isn't being affected by drink, cigarettes or recreational drugs is for you to avoid them completely, but if that's not realistic, then you need to be aware of the risks.

Let's start with drinking. As the latest research is unclear as to what constitutes a 'safe' amount of alcohol medical professionals currently advise that the best option is to avoid it altogether.

Smoking in pregnancy can stunt your baby's growth, but if you can't quit altogether, cut back as much as you can, as this will decrease the level of risk. Unfortunately, as medical treatments to aid quitting (like patches) aren't generally suitable for use in pregnancy (though some GPs will prescribe nicotine patches after the first trimester), it's a case of willpower, support and distraction – try joining a self-help group or taking up a yoga or meditation class to combat cravings, or ring the NHS pregnancy smoking helpline.

If you use recreational drugs, it would be wise to seek help from your GP in giving them up, as they may put your baby's health at risk. Help is also available from the National Drugs Helpline

Babyworld.co.uk members on smoking, drinking and drugs:

▶ *Han67 says:* 'My advice would be to use the services available – both NHS and private. Alternative therapies like hypnosis and acupuncture are worth investigating. Tackle one thing at a time, but if you're still finding it difficult then ask your GP for a referral to an appropriate practitioner.'

▶ *Ozz says:* 'It can be very hard to make these kinds of changes on your own. It helps if you have a supportive environment as well. If your partner continues to drink heavily when you are trying not to, that is going to make it much more difficult for you. The same applies to smoking and drugs. Men need to be sensitive to how difficult these kinds of changes are to make.'

▶ *Peta says:* 'I read lots of advice on whether or not to drink in pregnancy and decided in the end that it was a case of 'everything in moderation'. I didn't really fancy much in the first half of pregnancy anyway as I was frequently sick but as I started to recover it was nice to reward myself at the end of a hard week with a glass of wine. I'm sure those relaxed hormones whizzing round my system did baby more good than any harm the small amount of alcohol might have done!'

▶ *Mags01 says:* 'A friend of mine cut down to 10 a day, from about 25. The thing that annoyed me was the hard time her midwife and the support people gave her about those last 10. Smoking isn't good for you, it's worse for a baby and can cause all sorts of problems but as my midwife once said to me, any change is a good change and can help.'

See also:
Partner's attitude – page 126
Babyworld.co.uk link: **www.babyworld.co.uk/faq**

"I've been told it's important to exercise in pregnancy – but what's the best type of exercise, and can too much exercise harm my baby?"

KEEPING FIT AND EXERCISING

As with much of the advice on lifestyle changes in pregnancy, the key here is moderation. Exercise during pregnancy helps to keep your energy levels up, and women who are physically fit are better able to perform the hard work of labour and delivery.

That being said, pregnancy is not a time for extreme physical exertion. Pumping iron in the gym or marathon running are activities best reserved until after your baby is born. Good exercise is the kind that leaves you feeling slightly puffed and pleasantly relaxed – a brisk walk, swimming, yoga or gentle aerobic exercise are all excellent examples.

Moderate exercise is safe throughout pregnancy, though many women feel more able to exercise during the second trimester when early symptoms have calmed down and their bump is still quite small. Make sure you drink plenty of fluid before, during and after exercise and try to ensure you don't get too hot or short of breath. It's better to exercise regularly for short periods (around 20-30 minutes two to three times a week is plenty) than to have one major session each week.

Babyworld.co.uk members on keeping fit and exercising:

▶ *Brumb says:* 'When I was pregnant with my first child, I continued to cycle to work apart from a week near the beginning when my morning sickness got so bad that I felt as if I'd fall off the bike. I stopped when I was 6 or 7 months pregnant because I started to get SPD-like symptoms. I was concerned that cycling in pregnancy had brought it on, but was subsequently assured by my doctor that this was highly unlikely.'

▶ *Suki says:* 'I did yoga for a year before I fell pregnant, developing a love affair with it. I then did antenatal yoga when I was pregnant. It's great for getting your heart pumping but also for developing strength in all your muscles. It's great for women as there's a lot of emphasis on strengthening your core muscles; your pelvic floor, back and abdominal muscles.'

▶ *Mags01 says:* 'I think the second trimester is a good time to exercise and keep fit. I've always found that during the first trimester, I feel exhausted, sick and lethargic, and then during the final few months exercise is quite difficult with a huge bump and increasing tiredness.'

▶ *Ozz says:* 'I tend to do a lot of swimming and walking during pregnancy. I think it lifts your mood and prepares you well for childbirth. It's good that more classes are opening exclusively for pregnant women, as it's a good opportunity to meet other mums and share worries too.'

See also:
Blooming and boosted energy – page 80
Smoking, drinking and drugs – page 118
Relaxation techniques – page 138
Babyworld.co.uk link: **www.babyworld.co.uk/faq**

> "Since we found out I'm pregnant, I've been worried about having sex. What are the risks to my baby?"

SEX IN EARLY PREGNANCY

Many women worry about penetrative sex in pregnancy, whether it's the fear of orgasm bringing on premature labour, or the thrusting of the penis causing miscarriage. But there's no medical evidence that sexual activity in pregnancy does any harm whatsoever.

In extreme cases there are exceptions. If you have a tendency to miscarry, your GP might suggest you avoid intercourse for the first three months. If you have a history of premature labour, you might want to avoid intercourse later in pregnancy. If you have a low-lying placenta, your GP may suggest you avoid intercourse.

Just because you can have sex, that doesn't mean you have to. Levels of desire in pregnancy vary greatly, and while some women find their sex drive is heightened, others may feel too ill or too anxious to attempt sex at all. Men experience the same rollercoaster, some find the process of pregnancy sexually exciting, some are too fearful (or bashful) to have penetrative sex.

If there's a huge gulf between your desires and your partner's, it is vital to find a way to talk about this, as pregnancy is a bad time for either of you to feel unloved. There are many alternatives to penetrative sex (see below), all of which can help to maintain the essential intimacy of your relationship.

Babyworld.co.uk members on sex in early pregnancy:

▶ *Lupa says:* 'We stopped having sex when I was 10 weeks pregnant because I had a bleed. I was too scared to try for a good couple of months and then when I was ready for it, my husband wasn't. He loved my bump but just felt awkward about us having sex.'

▶ *Melrose says:* 'Our twins were the result of three years of infertility and ICSI treatment, so we were scared to indulge despite all the advice about it being OK. We just didn't want to risk the pregnancy. During the first trimester I felt too vulnerable (or rather the pregnancy was too vulnerable) and sick, and although I felt extremely sexy in the second trimester I feared that orgasms would trigger contractions.'

▶ *Megamum says:* 'I found our sex life soared while I was pregnant. My partner loved my changing body and I felt really confident about my shape. The only time it slowed was when he started to be able to see the baby moving through my stomach and it took him a bit of time and some different positions to get used to it.'

Variety adds spice

Pregnancy is a great time to experiment with new ways of making love. Pleasing each other without penetration can improve a couple's sex life. Here's a good example:

Begin with a bath by candlelight, then wrap your partner in warm towels and dry him or her, taking care over each part of the body. Rub your hands in warm lemon oil (avoid aromatherapy oils in early pregnancy unless you have consulted an aromatherapist) and gently stroke and massage your partner's limbs, back, shoulders and stomach. You may both feel like sleeping after this, or you may go on to achieve orgasm through touch.

See also:
Your changing appearance – page 116
Sex in later pregnancy – page 122
Partner's attitude – page 126
Babyworld.co.uk link: **www.babyworld.co.uk/faq**

"My sex drive has improved, but my appearance hasn't!
How can we have sex with a giant bump between us?"

SEX IN LATER PREGNANCY

As we've seen, sex in pregnancy will not cause direct harm to the baby (unless you have very rare and specific conditions – see page 122). But there are emotional considerations, you or your partner may feel awkward about sexual intimacy while your growing baby is such a tangible (and active) neighbour.

Again, there is a need to be open and honest with your partner about what you both want. The presence of a bump can be the perfect excuse to experiment with positions beyond the standard (and rather uncomfortable) missionary. Some couples prefer it if the woman is on top as this allows the woman to control the amount of penetration and keeps the weight off the bump. If the woman is on all fours with the man kneeling behind, this can allow more penetration. The 'spoons' position involves lying on your side with the woman's back towards the man's front, with him entering from behind. This keeps weight off the bump and makes penetration quite shallow, which some couples prefer during late pregnancy. It is a case of gentle experimentation and discussion.

Babyworld.co.uk members on sex in later pregnancy:

▶ *Mio says:* 'When you have a huge bump, it's undignified and often very humourous. But don't worry, labour is far more undignified. Nearing your due date, you will probably want to have sex loads to get baby out! This can really put your partner off as he feels he's being used for the hormones in his sperm. Tell him to get over it, after all, you're doing the rest of the work in the pregnancy and birth.'

▶ *TeriP says:* 'By the time I was up for some action again we had got out of the habit and he wasn't keen anyway. Not sure whether this was about the baby being right there, but suspect that it is more to do with body image and he just doesn't fancy me anymore. I try not to think about it, but feel very rejected. They say the woman is often the one who doesn't want sex. I have found this to be totally the opposite.'

▶ *Aggie says:* 'This is my third pregnancy and I have learned to accept the fact that my husband just doesn't fancy me when I'm pregnant. He is very honest and admits that whilst he loves me to bits and is amazed at my changing body and the impending baby, he just doesn't fancy me. I must admit that when I start to feel the baby move I find sex too strange, it's very off-putting feeling little wriggles and kicks when you're in the throes of lovemaking.'

An excellent excuse

While sex won't start labour unless the woman's body is ready, nipple stimulation and intercourse are natural ways to help induce labour in late pregnancy if your baby is overdue. The prostaglandins in semen soften the cervix, and hormones released by nipple stimulation encourage the uterus to contract. If you don't feel up to full intercourse, try a relaxing massage. Get your partner to focus on your breasts and clitoris. Orgasm may help nudge your body into labour and most women don't need penetration to achieve orgasm. If it doesn't work at least it will be fun trying.

See also:
Your changing appearance – page 116
Sex in early pregnancy – page 122
Partner's attitude – page 126
Bringing on labour – page 176
Babyworld.co.uk link: **www.babyworld.co.uk/faq**

"We both wanted this baby so much – why isn't my partner as excited as me? All he does is just moan about the extra work."

PARTNER'S ATTITUDE

In an ideal world you and your partner will sail through a flawless pregnancy in blissful accord. In reality, the various shocks, surprises and setbacks of pregnancy play havoc with the emotions of anyone who is emotionally involved.

As your partner isn't carrying the baby, he has no hope of understanding the physical demands of pregnancy. That also means he has no context for the emotional upheaval you're both experiencing. From his perspective, your relationship is changing and you are changing. His response to this may be to become more protective, or he may back away from an unfamiliar situation. Either response is natural, but may frustrate you and damage your relationship.

However much the balance of your relationship changes in pregnancy, it is vital to remain open and to discuss your feelings with your partner – and allow him to discuss his own valid concerns. The more he understands of the process, the better equipped he is to provide support when it is needed most.

Babyworld.co.uk members on their partners' attitude:

▶ *Mio says:* 'My partner is over the moon. I have never seen him so happy. He's been amazing, doing all the cleaning, washing and cooking.'

▶ *Kesie says:* 'I have had two miscarriages this year alone and so my partner refused to talk about the baby until I was at least 12 weeks. I felt really alone and depressed. We eventually had a big argument and I explained everything to him and also that the baby would thrive much more if I wasn't feeling so stressed. He has really started to turn around now, even to the point that when I was spotting he was more positive than me.'

▶ *McNeil says:* 'I think that it can be difficult for men during the early stages, as they can't really see anything going on externally and you are the one experiencing all the symptoms. Hopefully once you start to get a little bump and feel the baby move, he will feel a bit more involved.'

▶ *Parla says:* 'My partner is still 'celebrating' the news. He doesn't realise how much our life has changed already and I'm not even showing yet. He's going to get a shock when the baby comes along.'

▶ *NiaF says:* 'I am feeling pretty lucky. Mine won't let me lift or carry anything and is doing all the cooking and most of the cleaning. I am proud of him. We had a bit of a scare, some spotting and pain all day he kept me calm and smiling. To a certain extent I expect nothing less, though, I keep pointing out that he got me pregnant.'

▶ *Pip180 says:* 'My husband has had migraines, sickness, tiredness, the lot. I think it's just so he doesn't get landed with any extra duties.'

▶ *LaraP says:* 'My partner, despite the pregnancy being planned, had a real problem with my changing size. The ethos of being slim was in-built in both our lives and the stage where you fill out but don't look obviously pregnant was particularly difficult, made worse by comments on how awful I looked in particular clothes from my partner.'

See also:
Your changing appearance – page 116
Sex in early pregnancy – page 122
Babyworld.co.uk link: **www.babyworld.co.uk/faq**

"My mother-in-law said I must give my cats away, because they're a danger to me and my baby. Is there any truth in this?"

PETS AND BABIES

Pets suffer a pretty bad press when it comes to pregnancy, and the imminent arrival sometimes means the end of the road for a faithful friend. With no known risks to pregnant women from contact with dogs, it is normally cats that come off worse, as they can be the source of the harmful disease toxoplasmosis as well as having an unfair reputation for smothering babies in the cot.

While the smothering claim may be a bit of an urban myth, toxoplasmosis is a serious problem. Contracted from animal faeces or raw meat, this infection can also be carried by other animals such as sheep. A third of pregnant women are immune to the disease. For others, infection with toxoplasma can cause miscarriage in early pregnancy, and, unlike most infections, it can also cause problems later in pregnancy. However, many people who become infected have no adverse consequences for themselves or their babies.

Touching your cat does not expose you to the risk of toxoplasmosis. The only precaution you need to take is to either avoid the cat litter tray altogether or to wear gloves when emptying the litter tray. For the sake of hygiene, it is worth investing in a cat net for your baby's cot, and trying to keep all pets out of the baby's room where possible. For safety's sake, you should never leave your baby alone with your dog.

Babyworld.co.uk members on pets and babies:

▶ *FranK says:* 'We have bought a special cat net to put over the cot to stop the cat climbing in, also one for the carrycot. We decided against a Moses basket because I have images of not only the cat but also the three dogs climbing in for a kip!'

▶ *Peri89 says:* 'I'm going to resort to the good old 'squirting water on the cats from a bottle' trick! A few squirts and they won't go near the cot again. It worked on mine with the new sofa, and I'm going to try it again with all things baby, including the pram. It doesn't hurt them but they hate it, so it's worth a try.'

▶ *Suki says:* 'Buy a citrus repellant spray and spray it around the base of the basket – the cats hate it and will stay away.'

▶ *MeganD says:* 'I don't think there is any reason to get rid of cats – think how much your child will learn by having pets in the house, how to love, be gentle and considerate. Everything just needs a little tweaking to get everyone to live together smoothly.'

Cats and the cradle

Mags01's story:

'I've been a volunteer for Cats Protection for almost seven years. During that time I've fostered more than 300 cats, have had two babies and at the present time I have seven cats of my own.

'I've managed to bring up all of my children without any of them ever touching the cats' litter trays. It was always instilled into them that the litter trays were out of bounds. There is a risk of toxoplasmosis from cleaning the litter trays, but if you wash your hands with an anti-bacterial handwash afterwards there shouldn't be a problem. You are as likely to catch toxoplasmosis from unwashed fruit and vegetables or just by weeding the garden.

'We keep bedroom doors closed, so it's been easy for me to keep the cats away from the baby's cot. The cats never show much interest in babies. Babies are noisy, so my cats prefer to be elsewhere.'

See also:
Getting ill – page 98
Babyworld.co.uk link: **www.babyworld.co.uk/faq**

"My normal clothes are getting a bit tight – am I doomed to wear expensive, unattractive maternity clothes?"

MATERNITY CLOTHES

From decorator's dungarees to frilly-collared print dresses, everyone has their own image of what constitutes maternity wear. It's not always flattering, and the prospect of buying this 'utility' clothing doesn't always fill women with excitement.

But as with much of the pregnancy experience, maternity clothes have moved on in recent years – most high street retailers offer a selection in their larger stores, and the supermarket chains also have good and affordable ranges.

Borrowing or making maternity clothes can cut costs and can help you appreciate that this is a short, necessary phase in pregnancy. And you could always go shopping with the maternity clothes budget after the birth.

Babyworld.co.uk members on maternity clothes:

▶ *Peri says:* 'I found a good alternative to maternity trousers, which I was constantly having to hoist up. Yoga trousers! They are loose, comfortable and smart and they have a little adjustable tie at the top so that you can wear them over or under your bump.'

▶ *Lilkat says:* 'Borrow maternity wear if you can as this saves money. If you're expecting twins the chances are you'll outgrow your maternity wear. Get something with a massive expandable waist. You might look like Humpty Dumpty but you'll be more comfy.'

▶ *Tumla says:* 'Don't take the advice of shop assistants who tell you to just buy a large size in regular clothes. It's all very well buying a size 22 if you're usually a 14. It may well fit your bump, but it'll not touch you anywhere else.'

▶ *Pip 180 says:* 'I wasn't huge, so didn't get any maternity clothes until 16 weeks. Then I regretted not doing it sooner as all that elastic and Lycra is fabulous. Also, you won't want to wear jeans immediately after giving birth, something soft like jogging pants is better and more comfortable on bruised areas.'

▶ *Mags01 says:* 'If you know someone who can sew, you can get really lovely maternity sewing patterns and some fabric from most department stores or haberdashers. My mum made me a fabulous dress to wear to a wedding.'

▶ *Mio says:* 'I had painful trapped nerves as my bump got bigger and the only thing that helped was lying flat or holding my bump up. I bought every elastic/belly bra/belt I could find and each one went back as they were ineffective. I ended up buying a long piece of Lycra from a fabric shop and wrapping it round my bump as tight as possible and tying it underneath. Discreet under clothes, covered the whole bump and could be altered as I got bigger. A real relief from the pull at the top of my bump, it helped back ache too.'

▶ *CathO says:* 'Nearly new sales, table top sales, NCT sales, car boots – start trawling them whenever you can and ask anyone selling clothes if they have maternity stuff – it's really hard to sell on so you'll get it at knock-down price. Also put the word out a bit – when I've been pregnant I've had clothes from every angle without doing a thing!'

▶ *Lori P says:* 'Top tip for bras was when I had to move up a size (again) near the end of pregnancy I bought nursing bras and these were fine to start with after the birth too until I went and bought yet more in an even bigger size.'

See also:
Your changing appearance – page 116
Babyworld.co.uk link: **www.babyworld.co.uk/faq**

> **"There's so many things to buy, I don't know where to start. How does anyone afford the cost of a newborn baby?"**

WHAT TO BUY BEFORE THE BIRTH

Stop. Think carefully about the actual, day-to-day needs of a newborn baby. Then redo your shopping list. Take into account the fact that a baby needs somewhere to sleep, clothes to wear, some nappies and a changing area, a means of feeding and (if you're going out in the car), a properly-fitted car seat. Everything else can wait.

Of course, it's hard to avoid the temptation to treat your new arrival to a few special items, but be warned that, more often than not, the swing you've had your eye on for ages will prompt a screaming fit and will go into a cupboard never to be seen again. Postpone the shopping frenzy until you've become properly acquainted with your baby. You might just save yourself a fortune.

Babyworld.co.uk members on what to buy before the birth:

▶ *Tula says:* 'It is useful to have something that baby can sleep in during the day downstairs. We had a carrycot as part of our pram. I wouldn't buy 'proper' sheets, just use pillow cases over the mattress and then you can just turn them over when baby is sick.'

▶ *Aeon says:* 'Get a changing bag, but make sure your partner is happy to carry it (i.e. not too girly a design). My husband chose ours so we have one with lots of pockets. It's useful to have a detachable change mat and waterproof pocket for wet clothes/nappies. You don't really need a 'proper' change bag – a simple rucksack will do!'

▶ *GretaR says:* 'A playmat was good to have as something to lie on rather than carpet. Our son also loved a play gym. We didn't really bother with buying toys as we got loads as gifts and the baby wasn't interested for ages anyway.'

▶ *Kari says:* 'I wouldn't bother to get more than half a dozen vests and sleepsuits. You will get loads as gifts. Look for sleepsuits that have poppers down the front – you don't want to be rolling a baby over to mess about with poppers up their back, or having to persuade them that they want one put over their head.'

▶ *Mio says:* 'One thing I found totally indispensable was a baby sling – it made supermarket shopping so easy. I would advise people not to buy too much stuff to start with – newborns really don't need as much as you might think, and particularly with clothes, will grow out of them in the blink of an eye.'

▶ *Suse says:* 'If you're going to breastfeed, a nightie with poppers down the front might be useful (don't go with buttons as a hungry baby doesn't have the patience to wait). I would also recommend getting some cheap towels or muslin cloths to put on your changing mat as I found that if my baby weed while changing, she soaked her clothes, meaning a full change was needed.'

▶ *Pally says:* 'A girl I worked with bought tons of newborn nappies in all different brands – she then had a baby weighing 10lbs 12oz and ended up taking most of them back.'

▶ *Sigsi says:* 'I'd say if there's something you'd like to get and it's not essential for the first few days or weeks then I'd wait and try your baby in it before you buy, all babies are different and like different things.'

See also:
Packing for the hospital – page 172
Babyworld.co.uk link: **www.babyworld.co.uk/faq**

"I was waiting for a bus the other day and a woman in the queue started asking me all sorts of personal questions. When did my body become public property?"

DEALING WITH UNWANTED ADVICE

The weather, house prices and pregnancy – three subjects that everyone has an opinion on. So prepare for a verbal assault from taxi drivers, total strangers and work colleagues – as well as the inevitable advice from the previous generation of mothers.

It can be a real source of stress if you let it all get to you – and taking advice from someone who was last pregnant 30-odd years ago can be downright dangerous. Your best bet is to try and develop a personal 'advice filter'. Consider not just the advice, but the person offering it, and their track record as a parent. Then use or discard the advice as you see fit. If you keep an open mind, a permanent smile and a large reservoir of good humour you'll get through the experience – and you'll soon be offering advice to the next round of mums-to-be.

Babyworld.co.uk members on dealing with unwanted advice:

▶ *Kay07 says:* 'The best thing seems to be explaining your position once or twice and then, after that, listening politely and changing the subject as soon as possible...'

▶ *Maxi says:* 'The hardest part is having the confidence in yourself to do what you want rather than feel that you should follow other people. There is no one right way, just lots of different ways for different people. Life would be boring if we were all the same.'

▶ *Peta says:* 'By far the most infuriating advice is from well-meaning people with no knowledge or experience of the situation. The first topic that springs to mind for me here is homebirth. I was told by dozens of women (and a few men too!) that homebirth is possibly unsafe (or even actually dangerous). I had next to no support from friends and relatives; most were convinced I was doing something outlandish and terrifying, and tried to talk me out of it regardless of anything I tried to explain to them!

▶ *Marthasmum says:* 'There are some people who seem to think that not only should you listen to their (often misinformed) advice but that you should act upon it and who will challenge you about it if you haven't taken their advice to heart. I tend to try to avoid these people as much as possible!'

▶ *Teri says:* 'The wonderful thing about being a sixth time expectant mum is that almost no one attempts to offer you advice anymore. In fact it's me who is probably guilty of passing on advice without having been asked for it. It's driven by a desperation to pass on the few parenting tips which I know have genuinely helped me over the years and were probably only gained through making mistakes in the first place!'

▶ *Suze says:* 'I would weigh up the advice and think about their qualification to give it. Someone without any experience of raising children is little qualified to offer an opinion and on the whole should be smiled at and then ignored. A person with 30 years of experience with babies and children would however be worth listening too, babies are individuals but not aliens and what works for the majority could work for you too! Be open!'

▶ *Mika P says:* 'For some reason, I am public property. I wouldn't ever dream about putting my hand on someone's bump, unless they invited me to, but I am finding people are just coming up to me at work and putting their hand on my tummy!'

See also:
Worrying about the size of your baby/bump – page 88
Your changing appearance – page 116
Babyworld.co.uk link: **www.babyworld.co.uk/faq**

"I'd like to try some alternative remedies during my pregnancy. What are the benefits and risks?"

TRYING ALTERNATIVE REMEDIES

Midwife says: If you want to try alternative therapies and remedies in pregnancy, it's always best to consult a qualified practitioner. However confident you feel about using essential oils or other alternative treatments, you need to make sure that there is no risk from them to you or your baby.

Just because a product is 'natural', that doesn't mean it can't be harmful, and there are common remedies which should be avoided when you're pregnant, either because they're known to be harmful or, more often, because the effects of their use are unknown. An aromatherapist will advise which oils are safe to use in pregnancy. Homeopathic remedies are generally regarded as being safe for use by pregnant women, though it's best to consult a homeopath to find out which remedies would be most suitable in your individual circumstances.

Therapies like massage, reflexology, osteopathy, chiropractic and acupuncture may all provide some benefit in pregnancy. While it is essential to let the practitioner know that you are pregnant, these therapies are not harmful to you or your baby, although in some cases, the practitioner might not treat you in the first three months, just as a precaution. Their benefits may range from relief of certain symptoms – from aches and pains to nausea – to simply giving you the chance to relax and unwind.

Babyworld.co.uk members on trying alternative remedies:

▶ *Marthasmum says:* 'When my haemoglobin level slowly started to drop I took natural iron sachets to boost my iron levels. It worked and prevented a hospital birth – I was able to have my daughter at home as planned.'

▶ *Sal34 says:* 'I mainly used aromatherapy during my homebirth last time. I had one session with a qualified aromatherapist to discuss the best oils to use both in late pregnancy and during labour. I found the effect of the oils in the bathroom was similar to Entonox. They calmed me and helped me to breathe effectively.'

▶ *KP says:* 'I use a lot of complementary therapies both in my normal life and when I am pregnant. This pregnancy I tried acupuncture to try and help during the first 14 weeks when things were so bad that I literally couldn't move without vomiting and it definitely helped.'

▶ *LoriQ says:* 'I see a chiropractor regularly. This was particularly useful during my last pregnancy as my coccyx doesn't move or bend as it should during delivery. I think that I would have had much more pain with my lower back during pregnancy and birth had I not seen the chiropractor.'

▶ *Mum2B says:* 'I took arnica after my first caesarean section and found that I had no bruising or swelling, so plan to take it again for my next section. I have also had reflexology and found it very relaxing, but I don't know if it has any proven benefits for particular ailments.'

See also:
Getting ill – page 98
Relaxation techniques – page 138
Babyworld.co.uk link: **www.babyworld.co.uk/faq**

"As the weeks go by, I'm finding it hard to stay calm. Which relaxation techniques are safe to try in pregnancy?"

RELAXATION TECHNIQUES

Many techniques are safe to use in pregnancy, and some are so simple that you may not have thought of them as relaxation ideas at all. Here's some of the most effective:

Get out and about. Gentle exercise such as yoga is brilliant for relaxing the mind and toning the body. Swimming is another perfect exercise while pregnant – it keeps you toned and healthy, without being too strenuous. Even if you're starting to find walking harder, swimming should be easier as the water will carry your weight.

If you're on maternity leave, use the time to see friends and share the funnier side of your pregnancy experiences. Laughter is one of the body's best ways of relaxing. Fresh air, sunshine and a walk in the park are great quick fixes to relieve feelings of stress. And if you don't feel up for walking, then just sitting in the garden will help.

Chill out. A warm bath can do wonders. Add a few candles around the place and put on some relaxing music. Use meditation techniques to relax. Choose a time when you know you won't be disturbed and try to give yourself at least 30 minutes to meditate. Simply doing nothing is a good response to a busy and stressful life.

Have a treat. Take the time to relax over at least one delicious and nutritious meal a day. This is a great time to catch up with your partner and feel like a real person again. Visit a spa that offers treatments for pregnant women, buy pampering beauty products, treat yourself to some new jewellery or a haircut. Go on weekend breaks and make sure you take a holiday before the baby is born.

Babyworld.co.uk members on relaxation techniques:

▶ *MayaP says:* 'My top tip is pregnancy massage. I had several of these in my third trimester. They were £25 a go, but fabulous relaxation and time to prepare for what is coming by focusing on the baby. Next time round I would try hypnobirthing, which can be used to practice relaxation in pregnancy too.'

▶ *Sali says:* 'I slept as much as I could (lots of daytime naps at weekends), had relaxing baths in the evenings and kept exercising as long as I could including dance exercise classes until 34 weeks and lots of walking. I didn't realise how stressful I was finding work until I started maternity leave at 32 weeks but then I had a great time taking things slowly and working my way through my list of pre-baby tasks.'

▶ *Babs34 says:* 'I find that yoga is both fantastic for chilling you out and making you a nicer person and is also great for pregnancy in general, helping strengthen you up for the birth as well as relaxing you. Find a yoga for pregnancy class or contact a class and ask the teacher if she can tell you which postures not to do.'

▶ *ZemaP says:* 'Looking back I realise that more 'me' time was needed – more long baths, simply resting and listening to music. I should put everything else on hold and make sure I do that at least every day.'

See also:
Trying alternative remedies – page 136
Feathering the nest – page 158
Fear of labour – page 160
Handling the pain – page 186
Babyworld.co.uk link: **www.babyworld.co.uk/faq**

"I want to make the best use of my maternity leave – is it better to leave earlier, or work to the last minute and have more time with my baby?"

MATERNITY LEAVE

The rules regarding how long you can take for maternity leave and how much you will be paid vary to some extent depending on your circumstances and your company. You should ask your HR department or union representative for up-to-date information on the schemes in operation, as well as the rights and benefits that are available to you – as of April 2007, the new Work and Families Act is in force, extending the rights and leave options for working mothers. Check **www.dti.gov.uk** for the latest information. If you are self-employed, contact the benefits agency to see if you quality for Maternity Allowance.

You need to inform your employer of your intention to take maternity leave at least 15 weeks before your expected week of childbirth, though the leave can be taken any time from 11 weeks before the date your baby is due. Many women choose to wait until the latest possible date to start their leave, giving them more time with their baby. But that can be easier said than done, especially if your work involves a long commute or physically and mentally demanding tasks.

Depending on your circumstances, it might be advisable to give yourself enough time to rest and build up your energy levels before you start the hard work of labour and baby care.

Babyworld.co.uk members on maternity leave:

▶ *LoriP says:* 'I would recommend planning to leave work as late as possible, that way you have longer with your baby once it is born (if you are planning to go back to work), and also have less time before the birth to a: worry about it, b: over-shop and c: get bored waiting for the big event.'

▶ *Melrose says:* 'It would help if the better paid part of leave lasted longer. Luckily my company does give more than the basic otherwise I'd have been back a long time ago.'

▶ *Lilkat says:* 'When you are in early pregnancy and planning your maternity leave it sounds reasonable to work till 38 weeks or so. What you may not realise is that towards the end you get very tired, heavy and uncomfortable. Factor in travelling, and maybe looking after other children, and working till the last minute is not so appealing...I think about 35-36 weeks is a reasonable time to stop work, and it's really nice to have time at home before the baby comes to get organised, sleep, read and shop.'

▶ *TaraM says:* 'I fully intended to leave work at 34 weeks but when it got nearer the time I couldn't imagine going. I ended up staying until 38 weeks and wanted to do another week but they wouldn't let me because I worked so far away from home and they were worried I would go into labour there!'

▶ *Keli says:* 'I am self employed and was worried if I was entitled to anything. The good news is my claim for maternity allowance has been accepted so I have decided to take the full 26 weeks off as I actually end up better off.'

▶ *Maya says:* 'I am going to start my maternity leave at the start of 38 weeks but have held back two weeks holiday which I could take before then if I am struggling. I am finding it hard to know what to do for the best as I have no idea how I will feel – I cannot imagine the commute will be fun so maybe I will be tempted to finish earlier!'

See also:
Paternity leave – page 142
Feathering the nest – page 158
Babyworld.co.uk link: **www.babyworld.co.uk/faq**

> "How much time can my partner have off to help after the birth – and will he get paid for any of it?"

PATERNITY LEAVE

Paternity leave has always been the poor relation of maternity leave, but recent measures have attempted to address the huge gulf between fathers' and mothers' rights. Even so, most men who wish to spend quality time with their new baby without losing a lot of income tend to arrange a period of annual leave to extend their paternity leave period.

Until April 2007, new fathers who had at least 26 weeks service with their employer were entitled to two weeks paid paternity leave, which is approximately £108 a week (as at April 2006), or 90 per cent of full salary if that is less than £108 per week. The leave must be taken within 56 days of the birth. Currently, half of all businesses continue to pay full salary to fathers taking paternity leave.

As of April 2007, the Work and Families Act gives employed fathers a new right to up to 26 weeks Additional Paternity Leave, some of which could be paid if the mother returns to work. For the latest information on paternity pay and leave visit **www.dti.gov.uk**.

Babyworld.co.uk members on paternity leave:

▶ *BellaG says:* 'My husband was lucky as his boss let him have two weeks off on full pay. I know not everyone will be able to get that, but if your partner can take some leave it'll be worth it. I was in hospital for two weeks, so he took his leave when I came home. He looked after me basically – did the housework, shopping, cooking, and just allowed me to focus on feeding the babies. He also really enjoyed just spending time getting to know the babies and being involved in looking after them. He's a very hands-on dad and I think it was partly down to him taking paternity leave.'

▶ *Lilli says:* 'Dads don't get a great deal when it comes to the birth of their children and employers should be more supportive in my opinion. My husband says he's never felt so emotional, shocked and elated in his life and he is so glad he could be part of the 'baby-moon' rather than just having to carry on as normal at work.'

▶ *Mags01 says:* 'My husband managed to get almost a month off work and boy was I glad of it! I gave birth just after Christmas so my husband already had a week off over the Christmas period, he then had his paternity leave, his place of work gave him an extra three days and then he took two days' holiday which meant I got a whole lot of time with him at home. I think fathers should be given a month's paternity leave, it gives them time to bond with their child and be there during the hardest readjustment of your life.'

See also:
Maternity leave – page 140
Antenatal appointments – page 146
Babyworld.co.uk link: **www.babyworld.co.uk/faq**

"We booked our foreign holiday before we found out I was pregnant. Will I have to cancel it now?"

TRAVELLING WHILE PREGNANT

Many women travel abroad while pregnant and they encounter no problems. That doesn't mean travel is risk-free, or that you shouldn't take precautions, especially when flying or travelling to less developed countries. The most important thing is to be forearmed with information about the facilities at your destination and well covered by a travel insurance policy that covers pregnancy complications and the care of a pre-term baby – not all policies cover these.

The first major risk of travelling while pregnant is getting ill. Pregnant women have a higher risk of contracting malaria, and there are few anti-malarial drugs available during pregnancy. Vaccines are best avoided during pregnancy, but when the risk of the disease outweighs that of the vaccine, they should be administered in the second or third trimester where possible. Pregnant women need to take particular care over contaminated food and water as diseases like listeriosis, toxoplasmosis and hepatitis E can have serious implications during pregnancy. Take drinks with you to prevent severe dehydration from diarrhoea. This can also be harmful for the developing foetus.

When flying, take care to minimise the slightly increased risk of deep vein thrombosis that exists during pregnancy and just after delivery. Most airlines won't accept pregnant women on their flights after 32 weeks; although in certain circumstances this can be extended to 36 weeks with a doctor's note. Travel insurance is also difficult to arrange beyond 32 weeks. Any long-distance travel beyond this stage is best avoided.

Babyworld.co.uk members on travelling:

▶ *Keto says:* 'It may be worth having a chat with your GP regarding air travel as he can prescribe compression socks to reduce the risk of DVT. Make sure you have travel insurance and drink plenty of fluids on the plane and get as much rest as possible.'

▶ *Peri says:* 'If you are driving over a long distance, be aware that you may be tired, though this mainly applies to the first and third trimesters. Plan your journey accordingly, considering time of day, leaving extra time for stops – for rests and the loo!'

▶ *Maxime says:* 'Consider how your seatbelt fits – this applies to both driver and passenger, from around 2-3 months pregnant. The lap belt should be under the bump and the shoulder belt between your breasts. In the event of an accident, or even sharp braking, an unborn baby can be seriously hurt by the forces exerted by the seatbelt. In my last car, the belt refused to stay under the bump, so I bought a seat pad with an elasticated, velcro-fastened strap that holds the lap belt down in the correct position.'

▶ *Lupe says:* 'Quite a lot of train companies will give you a free upgrade to first class as long as you hold an annual season ticket. Usually you just need to contact their customer services department and ask for it.   They will most likely ask for a letter from your GP, company or midwife confirming your due date (or a Mat B1 form if you have one) and a copy of your season ticket.'

▶ *Tera says:* 'London Underground have a scheme where they will send you a badge (bump on board) so that people can see that you are pregnant. This is particularly useful for the early stages where you feel absolutely awful but don't look at all pregnant.'

See also:

Getting ill – page 98

Babyworld.co.uk link: **www.babyworld.co.uk/faq**

> "I've got my 'booking in' appointment in a few days and I
> haven't a clue what to expect? How should I prepare?"

ANTENATAL APPOINTMENTS –
WHAT TO EXPECT

Normally, a trip to your GP at the start of pregnancy will trigger your first antenatal appointment, which is often known as the 'booking visit' and usually takes place between 11 and 13 weeks. This could be at your home, at your GP's surgery, or at your local hospital, depending on your area. You will be seen by a midwife and possibly also by a doctor.

Unless you have ongoing problems, this visit will probably be the longest and most detailed you will have. You'll be asked questions about your medical history, as well as about any family history of medical problems. You will also be asked about previous pregnancies. Your blood pressure will be checked and you will be asked to give samples of blood and urine. Weight and height measurements may be taken and the midwife or doctor may feel your tummy to assess the size of your uterus. You may be offered a dating scan to confirm when your baby is due.

After this, you may have appointments every four weeks until 28 or 30 weeks, every two weeks until 36 weeks and weekly after that, although it's not unusual for them to be less frequent than this. Appointments are often also less frequent in second and subsequent pregnancies.

At your regular appointments you will have further chances to ask any questions and discuss any worries, your blood pressure will be checked and you'll be asked to give a urine sample so that it can be checked for protein and for the sugar levels. You may be weighed or checked over for swelling in case of pre-eclampsia. The midwife will ask to feel your tummy to get an idea of how your baby is growing and, after about 28 weeks, which way it is lying. From about 16 weeks the midwife will be able to listen to your baby's heartbeat. You may be asked to give another blood sample at an appointment between 28 and 36 weeks. This will be tested to see if you are anaemic. In some areas a glucose tolerance test is given at this time to women at high risk of diabetes.

Babyworld.co.uk members on antenatal appointments:

▶ *Sly78 says:* 'I guess I naively thought my midwife and GP would be as excited about the baby as I was. They weren't. They see pregnant women all the time. I found most of my antenatal appointments disappointing. My midwife often tried to reassure me but didn't. When I asked her about things I had read about on babyworld.co.uk or other sites, she said "you should stop reading things, it will only worry you".'

▶ *TeriP says:* 'My midwife was excellent and I had good continuity of care – I saw her for all my appointments. She did several home visits too towards the end of my pregnancy. I felt able to speak to her about anything that was worrying me.'

▶ *Lara90 says:* 'My first experience of antenatal care left me very disillusioned. My midwife was on maternity leave so I didn't see the same one twice. As they wouldn't be seeing me again not one of them seemed interested in me. If I wanted to ask any questions or needed advice etc, more often than not I got told to ask at my next appointment as that would be my 'proper' midwife but it never was.'

▶ *Sali2 says:* 'As I was carrying twins I had monthly consultant appointments. I only saw my named consultant once – and that was on the day I was admitted to hospital with pre-eclampsia. Before that I saw members of the consultant's team – all very nice, but I felt a bit confused each time I left the appointment as they gave confusing and conflicting advice with regard to how my labour and delivery would be managed.'

See also:
Meeting the midwife – page 148
Scans – page 152
Babyworld.co.uk link: **www.babyworld.co.uk/faq**

"I'm nervous about meeting the midwife. What if we don't get on – will I be stuck with her for my whole pregnancy?"

MEETING THE MIDWIFE AND ESTABLISHING A RELATIONSHIP

Midwives are your guide through pregnancy, and to a degree they can help to shape your experience. That may be a positive thing, or it may be a source of stress if you don't find yourselves seeing eye-to-eye.

Though you'll probably be assigned a midwife at your booking-in appointment, it's quite rare to have the care of one dedicated midwife throughout pregnancy and labour, as most operate in teams. This can make relationship-building hard, but it also gives you the option to switch midwives if you feel you're not getting the support you need.

The most important thing to bear in mind when approaching your relationship with the midwives is the need to be open and frank at all times. Don't worry that you are giving them too much information or taking up time with your worries. If something is causing you concern, the midwife is there to deal with it or allay your fears.

Babyworld.co.uk members on midwives:

▶ *Kat21 says:* 'With my fourth pregnancy I had a student midwife follow my pregnancy, labour and postnatal care as part of a case-study. It was a wonderful experience. I was able to build up a friendship with her and had the confidence to ask so much more than I would have from a stranger. It was reassuring to know there would be a familiar face at the birth and to have talked through the birth plan beforehand. The aftercare was excellent and it was possible for her to see small changes in my mood and offer support and advice – a stranger would not have picked those up.'

▶ *Sami says:* 'My advice is be on time for your first appointment and remember to take your notes, water sample and anything else that you have been asked for. I would also bear in mind the nature of a midwife's job and expect to have to wait, take a book, drink and snack. The best way to build a good relationship with you midwife is to be honest, and not to expect her to know what you want or need automatically. Asking for an explanation or information is the only way that she will know that you need it. It is essential to disclose everything to the midwife, she can't help appropriately if you fail to tell her something important!'

▶ *Peto says:* 'I think that in order to establish a relationship with a midwife (or any one else for that matter) you have to see them relatively regularly. What has always worked best for me has been to write down all the questions that I want to ask and to be as open and honest about my worries as possible.'

▶ *Barra says:* 'A lot of my friends don't feel comfortable telling their midwife about piles or think that it's too much trouble if they are worried about lack of movement. This is awful and in some cases can be dangerous. If you don't feel you have a good relationship with your midwife you should try and change the one you are seen by. You need to trust them and be able to tell them things that you probably wouldn't feel comfortable telling other people.'

▶ *Ollo says:* 'My relationship with the midwife during my last pregnancy just felt right. I loved each antenatal appointment as she was funny and a delight to talk to. I've requested her this time and though she is booked up I will find a way. She's the sort of midwife who will fight for me, believe in me, encourage and support me. The sort where I don't need to write a birth plan because I know she won't do anything I don't want.'

See also:

Antenatal appointments – page 146
Babyworld.co.uk link: **www.babyworld.co.uk/faq**

"What are my options when testing for genetic abnormalities – and what are the risks of the tests themselves?"

TESTS FOR IRREGULARITIES

Antenatal testing for irregularities is an emotive subject, not least because it may bring you face-to-face with a dilemma over termination. But for many women, particularly those in their mid-30s and above, it's something to be understood and thought through. Before making any decisions on antenatal tests the first thing to understand is the difference between a screening test and a diagnostic test.

A screening test – like a blood test or nuchal fold scan – estimates your risk of having a baby with a serious health problem such as Down's syndrome or spina bifida. For example, a blood test at 16 weeks may estimate your risk of Down's syndrome as 1 in 500. With just one chance in 500 that your baby will have Down's syndrome, you are far more likely to have a normal, healthy baby than a baby with a disability. Screening tests aren't conclusive, but the result may reassure you.

If you're still concerned, a diagnostic test can tell you for certain whether your baby has certain major health problems. The two most common diagnostic tests are chorionic villus sampling (CVS), a test for Down's syndrome and other genetic abnormalities, and amniocentesis, a test for Down's syndrome, other genetic abnormalities and spina bifida. CVS is normally carried out at 11-13 weeks, amniocentesis around 18 weeks. Both carry a small risk of miscarriage, estimated to be between 0.5 and 2 per cent.

Your midwife or GP can provide more detailed information on these tests, the risks and your options post-diagnosis.

Babyworld.co.uk members on tests for irregularities:

▶ *Peta says:* 'The way I see it, the tests – even just waiting for the results of a blood test – can cause undue anxiety. I would find it hard to come to terms with facing the possibility of an abortion on such grounds and so I knew that there was no reason to go down that route.'

▶ *KarliP says:* 'As I had a previous miscarriage and bleeding during this pregnancy, I had already decided that I was not going to risk losing a healthy baby – we would just have to find a way to cope if our baby was born with abnormalities. I think that if I had not already lost a baby and come close to losing this one, I probably would have chosen to have an amniocentesis.'

▶ *Maya says:* 'I decided that the only tests that were necessary were ones where something definite could be told and where positive action could be taken to prevent further problems. Testing is important but should be weighed up. What's it for? What can be done about it? Are you willing to consider a termination?'

Mandi09's story

'Our second daughter was born at 34 weeks as a result of placental abruption, and was diagnosed four weeks later with a chromosome disorder causing her to have a severe muscle weakness.

With our third pregnancy, the decision to have an amniocentesis was relatively easy, it was waiting for the procedure and then for the results that was hard. We had agreed that if there was a severe defect we wouldn't continue with the pregnancy as it wouldn't be fair on our existing children, or us, but not knowing was hideous.

It is incredibly personal, but for us having a second child with health problems and special needs was not really an option.'

See also:
Antenatal appointments – page 146
Scans – page 152
Babyworld.co.uk link: **www.babyworld.co.uk/faq**

"What scans will I be offered in pregnancy and what is the purpose of each scan?"

SCANS

Though this varies from area to area, scans are usually offered at 12 weeks to date the pregnancy and again at 18-22 weeks to check for anomalies of the baby. Some areas only offer a 12 week scan for first pregnancies, while other areas only offer the later scan in all circumstances. If you have specific concerns regarding your dates or scans, speak to your midwife or GP.

During the dating scan a sonographer (ultrasound operator) measures the length of the baby from the top of its head to the end of its bottom (known as the crown-to-rump length, or CRL). The sonographer looks up this length on a table or computer database which converts the length into a gestation, or number of weeks pregnant.

At the anomaly scan, the sonographer takes a more detailed look at your baby. Various measurements are taken to check that your baby's growth is 'on track'. Conditions such as cleft lip and palate, spina bifida, plus any abnormalities of the brain, heart and other organs may also be identified at this scan.

Further scans will generally only be offered if problems develop – for example with the baby's growth, his position in the uterus, the quantity of amniotic fluid or the position of the placenta. NHS scans are only offered if there is genuine clinical need. Although there is no conclusive evidence that scans in pregnancy cause harm to unborn babies, it cannot be said that they are absolutely safe. Although an increasing number of women choose to augment the NHS scans by paying for private scans in 3D or 4D, as a rule scans must be used with caution, and only offered to women when the clinical benefits outweigh the risk.

Babyworld.co.uk members on scans:

▶ *Lula says:* 'After a miscarriage first time round we paid for a private viability scan at seven weeks. It was the best money we could have spent just to have the reassurance that there was a little bean there with a beating heart. My 12 week scan was lovely. It was done by a midwife, who even let us video it. My 20 weeks scan was more clinical – it was done by a sonographer. But, once we started asking questions he was willing to talk more about what he was looking at. Later on I ended up having another 6-7 scans one every fortnight, because of complications.'

▶ *GH34 says:* 'There was something quite special and exciting/nerve-wracking each time I had a scan. It always took a long time to get all the measurements (I had monthly, then fortnightly growth scans). My first couple of scans (before 12 weeks) were trans-vaginal. The foetus at this stage is rather blobby looking, with teeny little limb buds. The 12 week scan (if offered) is a good one – it's a recognisable baby! The 20 week anomaly scan is the 'biggie' - all the important checks are done. The rest of my scans were purely to measure how well the twins were growing, and to check the placentas and amniotic fluid.'

▶ *MayaP says:* 'I feel nervous about exposing a baby to soundwaves that close up, even if the risks may be low, so I keep them to a minimum. I agree they are a fantastic medical tool and invaluable in many cases, but personally I limit them to only ones I feel are really necessary. I'm not sure if I'd have a dating scan if I get pregnant again, although from a peace of mind point of view it's a lovely scan – other than that I don't think it serves much purpose.'

See also:
Antenatal appointments – page 146
Tests for irregularities – page 150
Babyworld.co.uk link: **www.babyworld.co.uk/faq**

"Will we be told the sex of our baby at the 20 week scan? I'm not certain I want to know, but then again, it might be a chance to bond."

FINDING OUT THE BABY'S SEX

There's only one way to identify the sex of an unborn baby and that is to have an amniocentesis done around 16 weeks or chorionic villus sampling (CVS) done around 10 weeks. In these tests, cells from the baby are analysed and the sex of the baby is identified.

Development of the genitalia of a foetus happens in the 10th and 11th weeks of pregnancy, so it is theoretically possible to have an idea of the sex of the baby from a scan after this time. But it's rare for even a clear scan to be 100 per cent certain, and for this reason many units will not tell parents the sex of the baby.

This necessarily cautious approach is partly motivated by a desire to avoid the emotional problems that can arise when parents are expecting one sex and the baby is born with the other. This can have a profound effect on the bonding process and may even be a contributing factor to more long-term problems such as post-natal depression.

Babyworld.co.uk members on finding out the baby's sex:

▶ *Kari says:* 'Our hospital has a sign up saying that they did a recent survey of people they'd scanned, and they were correct 96 per cent of the time. I can see how easily a mistake could be made. We could see something bobbing around when our son was scanned, but couldn't get a full frontal. So it could have been a penis – or his hand, or a bit of cord... We were told he was 'probably' a boy, but they couldn't be sure.'

▶ *LoriP says:* 'We decided to find out at the scan. This is because I suffered from post-natal depression last time and in a bid to try and 'bond' with my baby before birth I wanted to be able to have a name for him/her and be able to buy gender-specific things for them. We are having a little boy. When we talk about him, we use his name. It has also been a good way to help prepare our daughter. She knows she is going to have a little brother, so, she is also 'bonding' with him before he comes.'

▶ *Gio says:* 'We had a private scan at 23 weeks and discovered we were having another girl. Knowing we were having another girl allowed us to prepare physically and emotionally, and didn't reduce the excitement at all.'

▶ *Suki says:* 'We found out the sex at the 20 week scan and later had it confirmed at a private 4D scan. For me, I think it helped me bond with him before he was born. It also helped immensely with the practicalities – we didn't need to buy green and yellow clothes.'

▶ *Mags01 says:* 'I did ask with my daughter but they couldn't see so we had a surprise. I'm glad now that we didn't know as I was convinced I was having a boy so it was a fantastic surprise to have a baby girl.'

▶ *LiaMC says:* 'WARNING! Sometimes they get the scan wrong. We found out we were having a girl so I went and bought all these lovely pink dresses and decorations and all kinds of girly things, and we had a boy instead. I had imagined my little girl, and bonded with her – and for a while I found it really hard to equate the newborn boy I had with my ex bump. I will not be finding out next time, as I felt so confused and guilty about it all.'

See also:
Tests for irregularities – page 150
Scans – page 152
Babyworld.co.uk link: **www.babyworld.co.uk/faq**

"Is it vital for me to attend antenatal classes? If so, what are my options?"

ANTENATAL CLASSES

It's not essential to attend antenatal classes, and many women find the information in the classes repeats a lot of what they've read in books or on websites like Babyworld.co.uk. However, they are still extremely useful, both as an information source and as an opportunity to meet other parents-to-be.

Antenatal classes run by the NHS tend to offer more basic advice and support, though they differ from region to region. Classes run by the NCT (National Childbirth Trust) are often more structured and offer more detailed support. You have to pay for these classes and places are often quite limited, so early booking is advised. Alternatively, Babyworld.co.uk offers 'virtual' antenatal classes.

In addition to these classes, it is well worth seeing if your hospital offers a tour of the maternity unit, and if there are workshops available for breastfeeding and post-natal support.

Babyworld.co.uk members on antenatal classes:

▶ *Gio says:* 'I had NHS classes and they weren't bad – they went through the late stages of pregnancy, what happens when you go into labour, tour of the labour ward, a little bit of breathing, reminders to do your pelvic floor exercises every week What I could have done with was some sort of 'baby-handling' course because we had no experience of babies. I'd also recommend attending a breastfeeding workshop.'

▶ *KathM says:* 'I'm a volunteer for the NCT – their classes are worth doing as you have access to breastfeeding counsellors, you get more one to one help and you can make good friends and phone the antenatal teacher if you need any more advice. The NCT do refresher courses as well.'

▶ *Tula says:* 'I was given the forms for the NHS classes at my booking-in appointment. I had such a lot of paperwork to take in at that appointment, I very nearly missed them! Nothing has been said to me by anyone since, so it was pure luck that I spotted the forms and sent them off to apply for my place.'

▶ *Kayla says:* 'Later on in pregnancy, I enjoyed chatting online to the ladies in my babyworld.co.uk antenatal club – it was reassuring to hear from others in the same position.'

▶ *Sylvian says:* 'Don't worry too much about not going to classes. We only had them in the last few weeks here and I know a few people who missed them altogether. They still managed to have healthy babies! It's great for meeting people locally but I found my post-natal classes better for that. Everyone was a bit too fazed in the antenatal class to bond.'

▶ *PamPup says:* 'All I can say is, ask lots of questions if you have any. And write them down, otherwise you'll forget it all.'

▶ *Maxi says:* 'What I am finding far more useful now is yoga for pregnancy classes; there you learn all the breathing and relaxation and positions, and it chills you out big time. Every position feels so good, all those aches and pains just go.'

▶ *Cebo says:* 'Our hospital did a separate tour of the maternity unit which I found helpful. They told us useful things like where to park, where exactly to go on arrival, and what to bring. We saw a delivery room and various bits of equipment, the operating theatre, the post-natal ward and also the special care baby unit. It was all really useful.'

See also:

Babyworld.co.uk link: **www.babyworld.co.uk/faq**

> "With nothing else to do I can't stop tidying the house. I've dusted three times today already. Am I going mad, or is this my nesting instinct kicking in?"

FEATHERING THE NEST

Whether it's simply a desire to 'clear the decks' before the new arrival, to get organised in advance of post-natal chaos or something more spiritual, the nesting instinct does seem to exist for many women.

There's nothing wrong with keeping active in the countdown to labour, as long as you're not putting any undue stress on yourself or your baby. But it's also fine to rest and take things easy at this time. Experts recommend that your baby sleeps in the same room as you for at least the first six months, so there's no rush to decorate the nursery, and as for cooking and cleaning – well, that's what visitors are for.

If your family and friends are itching to help, now's the time to be selfish, rest, build up your energy reserves and let them take the strain of ironing, cleaning and tidying. Your hard work is just around the corner, and you need to be in a calm, relaxed and balanced state of mind.

Babyworld.co.uk members on feathering the nest:

▶ *MinaK says:* 'In early pregnancy the idea of the so-called 'nesting instinct' made me literally cackle with laughter. Fast forward seven months and you find me on my hands and knees scrubbing and tidying the kitchen from top to bottom. The baby's room is cleaned, tidied, rearranged and cleaned over and over again even though I know he won't be in there for around six months after he's born! It happened without me having any conscious thought, I just suddenly started doing it. I suppose I also wanted as little as possible to do once he was here so I could spend my time with him.'

▶ *Sali says:* 'I know it's really boring but before the new arrival makes an appearance try to cook and freeze a few meals in advance – I didn't want to spend the first couple of weeks chained to the kitchen, and neither did I want to eat junk every day.'

▶ *Pip180 says:* 'The last month or so, I would scrub my house from top to bottom most days, including scrubbing my skirting boards. I just couldn't seem to get things clean and tidy enough which is definitely not my usual nature.'

▶ *Lupo says:* 'No nesting instinct here at all. I think I swapped it for a sleeping instinct. I found it really hard to shift my bum in the last couple of months so did the absolute bare minimum of everything. Thank goodness I have a domesticated hubby!'

▶ *Lilkat says:* 'Everyone says save it for when you've had the baby, but I say rest as much as possible when you're pregnant. Despite the 'sleep when baby sleeps' advice you get after the birth, very few women actually follow it. If it is your first pregnancy, enjoy plenty of time just lying around tuning into your baby-belly. You don't get a medal for rushing around like a mad thing and the rest is good for your health and the baby's.'

▶ *Hili says:* 'It never seemed to happen to me, in fact the few days just before my son was born I almost wanted to hibernate. I had all these things that still needed doing and no inclination to do them at all, just an urge to lie around the place, reading or dozing. I think my body was conserving my energy for the big event. I did some very hurried and last-minute cleaning and ironing in the early stages of labour though, all the while cursing the fact I hadn't done it before.'

See also:
What to buy before the birth – page 132
Babyworld.co.uk link: **www.babyworld.co.uk/faq**

"I'm excited about the fact that I'm going to meet my baby soon – but I'm terrified about the labour. How can I ease my fears?"

FEAR OF LABOUR

As the big moment gets closer, it's entirely natural for your thoughts to turn to the labour. For first-time mums it's a journey into the unknown and your concerns might range from fear of the pain involved to a more general worry about losing control, or being so exposed and vulnerable in front of strangers. You may worry about how your partner will act at the birth, or how he will feel about you afterwards. You may worry about complications and interventions.

Forewarned is forearmed, so if you have concerns, find out more information from decent, authoritative sources like magazines, books, videos and established websites. Steer clear of out-of-date information (which can include the 'wisdom' of the older generation) and scare stories about other people's labours. Those are their experiences. Yours will be different.

Antenatal classes are another source of good information, and will teach you practical skills such as relaxation and using alternative positions. Good classes also provide an opportunity to talk about your worries, and make new friends.

For a few women, the fear of childbirth is sufficiently overwhelming for them to want to give birth by caesarean rather than face normal labour. This fear is known as 'tocophobia'. Talking to your midwife or doctor about your fears may help, or they could put you in touch with an expert counsellor. As a last resort, arrangements may be made for your baby to be born by caesarean.

Babyworld.co.uk members on fear of labour:

▶ *Karli says:* 'I found that the best way to cope with the fear of labour, was to convince myself from the very beginning that it would be a breeze! I know it sounds daft, but having a positive attitude really helps. I would tell everyone who asked "Aren't you scared?" – No, of course it's going to hurt, but it'll be a 'good' pain as I'll have my baby at the end of it. Anyone who tried to tell me labour horror stories would be told "I'd rather not hear this, as my labour is going to be wonderful".'

▶ *MayaP says:* 'Bear in mind that we're culturally conditioned to expect labour to be a horrendous experience. In a lot of cultures it's viewed in a completely different light and as a result there's very little fear involved.'

▶ *Pip180 says:* 'Throughout pregnancy I thought about labour along the following lines: it's going to happen, there's not much I can do about it and it's the only way of getting a baby; loads of people have done it and survived, therefore there's no point worrying about it; afterwards I won't remember much anyway, so it doesn't really matter either way. I did NHS and NCT antenatal classes and read up, but consciously decided not to worry about labour.'

▶ *Hari says:* 'I had a huge panic around 32 weeks about whether I'd get the baby out, but that passed. And by the last couple of weeks I couldn't care how he was coming out – as long as he did. I truly didn't believe anyone who said not to worry as you don't remember the pain, but in my case it's true. I only remember the lovely things.'

See also:
Antenatal classes – page 156
Handling the pain – page 186
Labour – page
Babyworld.co.uk link: **www.babyworld.co.uk/faq**

"Do I have to give birth in my local maternity unit? The facilities there seem limited, so I'd love to have another option."

CONSIDERING DELIVERY OPTIONS

In most cases it is up to you where and how you have your baby – at home, in a birth centre, in the local maternity unit, or in another hospital. Your place of birth is one of the biggest factors affecting how well your birth goes, so it's a crucial decision. We'll look at home birth in more depth elsewhere – see page 164 – but the following are some of the other alternatives to a standard hospital delivery:

Water birth. This is an increasingly popular delivery option – it is particularly flexible as you can do this at home, in a hospital, or as part of a 'low-tech' delivery at a birth centre. If you want a water birth in a hospital, there are practical factors that need to be considered. There may not be any facilities at your chosen hospital, the pool may be in use when you go into labour or there may be a shortage of midwives trained in water birth. Practices in different hospitals vary, but if there are factors which complicate the birth in any way, midwives will probably advise caution in the use of the pool. In certain circumstances they might be happy to support a woman labouring in water, but then help her out of the pool for delivery.

Birth centres. These provide a more relaxed and 'low-tech' approach to birth. Some offer facilities that hospitals cannot, such as better access to birthing pools and complementary remedies. Birth centres can offer 'conventional' pain relief such as gas and air and sometimes, but not always, pethidine. They don't offer all types of pain relief, in particular epidurals, and cannot conduct assisted deliveries. If your baby is showing signs of distress, you will almost certainly be transferred by ambulance to the nearest hospital. Most birth centres will only accept women who have not had complicated pregnancies and, therefore, are unlikely to have problematic labours.

To get a good idea of the different atmospheres of a hospital delivery suite and a birth centre, you should visit both and feel free to ask them any questions, it's best to go into this decision as forewarned as possible.

Babyworld.co.uk members on considering delivery options:

▶ *Suki says:* 'I decided to have my baby at a midwife-led unit. I wanted a water birth and they have 100 per cent water birth trained midwives. My experience was amazingly positive. Although the birth and labour were much more traumatic than my first pregnancy due to the position of the baby, my whole labour experience was so much better. I can't recommend a water birth enough, it's incredible how the water helps to reduce the pain.'

▶ *BabsD says:* 'I laboured in the birthing pool with my first but didn't deliver in there. I got to the hospital when I was 8cm dilated and so they said get straight in. I have to say it was lovely being in there, sucking on the gas and air with each contraction. The room was dark and quiet with the radio on in the corner and I had a lovely midwife.'

▶ *Mel23 says:* 'The midwife at the birth centre showed my husband how to massage my back to help ease the pain and she encouraged and assisted him. I know that this really helped him feel part of the process.'

▶ *ToniK says:* 'I think birth centres are an excellent idea, allowing women and their partners who are not entirely comfortable with the idea of home birth to still give birth in relaxed surroundings, free to move around and labour normally.'

See also:

Home birth – page 164

Babyworld.co.uk link: **www.babyworld.co.uk/faq**

> **"I'm keen on a home birth, but I've heard it's not a good idea for first pregnancies. Is this true – if so, why?"**

HOME BIRTH

There are no hard and fast rules preventing a woman from having a home birth – whether it is her first pregnancy or her fifth. Some women encounter resistance to the idea because of the personal views of a doctor or midwife, but it is your right to demand a medical reason for the refusal of a home birth.

Certain conditions must apply to ensure the health of mother and baby, given the lack of specialist medical equipment associated with this type of delivery. If you go into premature labour (before 37 weeks) or if the baby is in distress, or if there are other specific medical conditions concerning the midwife, you will be advised not to have a home birth. Otherwise, the option should be made available to you, and full support should be given.

Your midwife will have a list and plenty of guidance concerning the items needed for a home birth. All the midwifery equipment will be supplied by your local hospital, so there is no need to worry about bowls, jugs, cotton wool or the like. To protect the area where you'll give birth, you may wish to use old shower curtains as well as plenty of towels or sheets.

It's also important to have access to a telephone and focused lighting – a torch or table-top light is fine. You will also need some extra support around the house for a minimum of a week (ideally two or three) afterwards. Rest and time to get to know your new baby and establish breastfeeding is absolutely vital.

Babyworld.co.uk members on home birth:

▶ *Gio says:* 'Despite extensive research proving homebirth to be at least as safe as hospital birth, there still seem to be many people who insist that childbirth is dangerous and should be viewed as a medical procedure. Many of the problems women experience in hospital may not have happened had they given birth in natural surroundings without interference, without lying flat on a bed attached to monitors or drips.'

▶ *Keli says:* 'I don't think it's taken into consideration how vital the birth experience is to women and their wellbeing. A positive birth experience can lead to better bonding, a better chance of breastfeeding successfully and lower rates of post-natal illness. Home births are far cheaper than hospital births for the NHS, and have so many benefits.'

▶ *MaraD says:* 'I've opted to be under the care of the hospital but have decided that I'm going for a home water birth – my midwife is aware of this, and it's on my notes. They support home water births and I'm getting excited at the prospect.'

▶ *Mum2B says:* 'I was lucky last time that I found an NHS midwife able to support me with a home birth but I know from experience that many women have to go private to achieve this. A good birth experience is so important. I hate it when people say that all that matters is a healthy baby. Yes, that is vital – but so is a good birth experience.'

▶ *Tela says:* 'First time round I wanted a home birth but the midwife and GP wouldn't hear of it and I was booked for a hospital birth. I didn't know that in fact it's my choice where I give birth and I allowed the medical professionals to take over.'

See also:

Considering delivery options – page 166

Babyworld.co.uk link: **www.babyworld.co.uk/faq**

> **"I've heard a lot of pros and cons for medical pain relief in labour – but what are my options?"**

CONSIDERING PAIN RELIEF OPTIONS

It's a good idea to read up on pain relief options before the birth; even if you are resolute that you won't have any, or that you'll only use a certain option, it is always possible that you will change your mind when in labour. Not all options are available in all places, so check what you can access in your chosen delivery venue. It is also a good idea to be aware of the options for non-medical pain relief, including alternative or complementary therapies (see box).

There are several choices to make regarding medical forms of pain relief – Pethidine, TENS, Gas and Air (Entonox) and epidurals (both traditional and mobile). Each has its advantages and disadvantages, so talk through your options with your midwife. The right choice will depend in part on how far into labour you are, and how quickly labour is progressing. Your midwife will do an internal examination to see how dilated your cervix is and this will help you decide which form of pain relief is most appropriate.

Babyworld.co.uk members on considering pain relief options:

▶ *PiaD says:* 'My epidural was wonderful. The pain didn't go away entirely – but it was bearable, and I could feel enough to know when to push.'

▶ *Katsmummy says:* 'I had an epidural with my first and would not have one again. I found I had bad headaches for ages after and backache for quite a while. My labour was long and I could not feel to push so I ended up with forceps. I was up and about four hours after but my legs were hard to control.'

▶ *Mio says:* 'I had an epidural because I had high blood pressure and it brings it down. And I must say my experience of it was brilliant and I would definitely have it again. Whilst they were putting it in I was on the gas and air so don't remember feeling anything.'

▶ *Wildchild says:* 'I used TENS and gas and air last time. I'll definitely use TENS this time. It is quite fiddly to put on so it helps to have a practice before the real moment comes.'

▶ *Suki says:* 'I hired a TENS machine in my last pregnancy, and used it in the early stages of established labour. My baby had his back to my back and I had awful back pain. I found the Tens to help quite a bit, in fact I refused to let them take it off me until the very last moment before my epidural was sited.'

▶ *MayaP says:* 'I managed with a TENS machine – which I don't think did anything for the pain but was useful to have something to focus on – and gas and air. I thought the gas and air was brilliant once I'd got used to it, the midwife had to prise it away from me!'

New labour, old remedies

Many women choose to use complementary therapies such as acupuncture, hypnosis and aromatherapy to help them cope with labour. For some women these therapies are very useful, and they need no other form of pain relief. For other women these therapies work best alongside mainstream medical forms of pain relief. It is very important that whoever you go to for advice is properly qualified and affiliated to one of the recognised bodies that monitor the delivery of complementary therapies.

See also:
Handling the pain – page 186
Labour – page 180/188
Babyworld.co.uk link: **www.babyworld.co.uk/faq**

"I've been encouraged to write a birth plan, but I'm not sure where to start. What should I include, and will anyone actually read it?"

WRITING A BIRTH PLAN

Writing a birth plan is a very personal experience. Some women feel that a detailed plan is too prescriptive and may lead them to be disappointed if the labour doesn't go as planned, whereas others feel it is essential to set out their aims and ambitions for labour as a solid starting-point for the experience. While it's true that labour rarely progresses along imagined lines, it is also fair to say that a birth plan is an asset, even if it just helps you and your birth partner feel more relaxed during labour.

When composing your birth plan, try to keep it as brief and easy to read as possible. Remember that the midwives and other medical staff attending your labour will not have the time to study a lengthy document, so using bullet points will get your message across more effectively.

Topics to consider for your birth plan include pain relief choices, positions for labour, your opinion on interventions, monitoring or episiotomy, your views on assisted delivery and caesarean birth, whether you want skin-to-skin contact with your baby immediately, whether you want your baby to have a vitamin K injection, and whether you want an injection to speed up the delivery of the placenta.

Start thinking about these topics and any others you want to mention as early as possible and discuss your plan with your midwife. The more discussions you have with medical staff prior to labour, the better the chance that you will create a realistic and effective birth plan.

Babyworld.co.uk members on writing a birth plan:

▶ *Luka says:* 'The key is to be flexible and clear. It needs to be easy for a midwife to pick up and grasp the key points, as the shifts change and they are often rushed. If it is all dense paragraphs they may not take it in quickly enough.'

▶ *MandiP says:* 'Prioritise what your most important ideas are and make sure they are clear. One of my friends did hers on a flip chart and her husband stuck it to the delivery room wall -it had pictures too! Don't be afraid to re-write it if circumstances change. Once we knew I was going to be induced we wrote a fresh birth plan for induction.'

▶ *Keylo says:* 'Things can be misinterpreted. We said we wanted people to be quiet at the actual birth and dimmed lights. I couldn't feel how to push because of the epidural and what I really needed was people cheering me on, but the midwives were whispering because that was what I had requested. This was quite unnerving, as I thought they were talking about me and saying I couldn't do it! Once I lost confidence then forceps were needed.'

▶ *Gio says:* 'We took lots of time writing my birth plan, making sure it was flexible and using bullet points to make it clear and easy to read at a glance. When the time came it all went to pot. I had specifically stated I did not want pethidine, but as I had to be on my back on the bed, when I was in a lot of pain I kept trying to get up. The midwife gave me a shot of pethidine – without even asking me – to make me lie still. That really upset me.'

See also:
Choosing and briefing a birth partner – page 170
Babyworld.co.uk link: **www.babyworld.co.uk/faq**

"I love my husband dearly, but I'm worried he might not be much use at the birth and I really feel I'm going to need support. What can I do?"

CHOOSING AND BRIEFING A BIRTH PARTNER

The world has come a long way from the days when men were banned from the delivery suite. Nowadays few men miss the birth of their children, but as your partner is emotionally involved in your well-being and in the whole process, he may not necessarily be the right person to rely on at a time of great stress.

Some women feel more comfortable having support from a female relative or friend. It's certainly a good idea to choose a birth partner who knows you well, and ideally one who has experienced childbirth themselves. Bear in mind that you can have support from more than one partner, so it might be worth combining care from the father-to-be with the cooler head of an experienced mum.

Doulas are professional birth partners, and are an excellent option for women who feel they have no other suitable choices, but who need a little more support in labour.

Babyworld.co.uk members on birth partners:

▶ *Sali says:* 'My birth partner was my husband. He came to all of my antenatal classes with me, and possibly paid even more attention. We talked about things that were brought up in the antenatal classes, and he also read large parts of the books I had.'

▶ *LoriP says:* 'When I was planning my third labour, I had a frank chat with my husband and told him I needed his pro-active support to help me achieve the birth I wanted if I was unable to communicate clearly during labour. He was a big help to me as moral support, but he still didn't really put my views forward and tended to appear quite intimidated by the midwives, but luckily I was so relaxed that I was able to communicate well myself, and said what I did and didn't want.'

▶ *Tina21 says:* 'You are allowed to have more than one person with you and this can be very useful. All you really need is someone who can keep a level head. It can be very useful to have more than one birth partner so that they can actually take turns to be with you and get some rest. Labour is hard work for the person giving birth, but it's also hard work for the birth partner. It can be very emotional and very difficult for someone to watch the person they love in a lot of pain.'

▶ *Suse says:* 'Briefing your birth partner is important. They need to know what things you absolutely do not want and also what things you are flexible on. I think it's easier if your birth partner is someone who knows you well enough to be able to see if you are about to make a decision you will later regret and to be able to persuade you against it if this is the case. My husband and I have talked about what happened at my previous birth, what we learnt from it and we have been through my birth plan together so that he knows what I want and don't want.'

▶ *Maya says:* 'Keep an open mind as you may change it several times especially if things aren't going to plan. Ask for everything and every decision to be explained to you thoroughly. Choose a birth partner who will back you up and fight your corner if needs be as you may not be feeling you have the energy for it when in labour.'

See also:
Babyworld.co.uk link: **www.babyworld.co.uk/faq**

"I haven't got a clue about what I need to take with me to the hospital. What is provided and what should I bring from home?"

PACKING FOR THE HOSPITAL

Packing the hospital bag is one of those things everyone intends to do in an ordered and organised environment. But when reality bites some women are still left with a mad scramble to throw a few bits together in the pauses between contractions. Or worse still, they rely on their husbands to do it.

The resulting chaos won't cause any major problems – especially not in the age of 24-hour shopping – but it might add another dimension of stress to an already fraught environment. So try to get organised early, and think carefully about the essentials you'll require. Even if you're hoping to be in and out within hours, it makes sense to plan for a two or three day stay. And don't make assumptions about facilities provided by the hospital, they are likely to be basic, so you'll feel much more comfortable if you've got your own clothes and towels to hand.

You will almost certainly need to use maternity pads during the days immediately after the birth, so it would be a good idea to include some of these in your bag.

Babyworld.co.uk members on packing for the hospital:

▶ *Kia says:* 'I used two small bags for my stay as storage space is usually quite limited in hospital and I knew a small bag would fit under the bed. When I packed the bags I put a luggage label on each which said what the bag was for and also anything that needed to go in at the last minute (like hair and toothbrushes etc.). The theory was that my husband would be able to throw in the last few things if I couldn't.'

▶ *Peto says:* 'Lip salve is really useful. The gas and air made my lips really dry! Also in some of the baby shop catalogues there are useful checklists. Might be worth a look if you're unsure what to pack.'

▶ *MinnieP says:* 'If you're planning on staying in overnight pack some food! The 16 hours between dinner and breakfast go very slowly.'

▶ *Suki says:* 'Pack maternity pads – the staff at the hospital moaned about the fact that I hadn't brought any – but I did pack my bag two days before I went into labour so it was rather hurried.'

▶ *LornaW says:* 'Books, magazines, maybe an mp3 player or walkman will all be included next time round. And comfortable, loose clothes to go home in. Even if you have a digital camera, take a disposable one just in case, because batteries can (and most likely will) run out.'

▶ *MaraMW says:* 'I really thought disposable knickers were ace. I would never leave a pair of cotton knickers in the hospital bin and didn't want to roll them up and put them back in my bag when visitors were there. I agree they are not the nicest underwear I've owned but I loved them at the time. Do get a size bigger than usual though.'

▶ *Mum2B says:* 'I thought disposable knickers were rubbish and very uncomfortable. Also, I had a c-section and they rubbed my scar in a horrible way. I bought some value pants (they go up to big sizes!) and threw them away when I stopped bleeding.'

See also:
Bleeding after the birth – page 204
Babyworld.co.uk link: **www.babyworld.co.uk/faq**

> **"My midwife says my baby's head is engaged – what does this mean exactly, and am I going to be in labour soon?"**

BABY'S HEAD ENGAGES

The baby's head is 'engaged' when the widest part of the head has moved down into the pelvis – that is, when less than half (2-3/5) of the head can still be felt by the midwife (or palpated, in medical speak) abdominally.

The timing and significance of engagement depends on several factors. Firstly, women expecting their first baby tend to have firmer abdominal muscles, so their babies may be gently eased down into the pelvis during the last four weeks of pregnancy. A second or third baby may not become engaged until labour starts.

It also depends on the position in which your baby is lying. If your baby is 'posterior' (with his back against your back), then his head will not be in the best position to fit into the pelvis during pregnancy. It may take some strong uterine contraction to ease him downwards.

Thirdly, the shape of your pelvis is a factor. Some women – generally those of African descent – find that their babies do not descend into the pelvis until labour starts. It is also important to remember that a baby may move in and out of the pelvis, especially if he still has plenty of room. Your baby may well stay at 4/5 until you start having contractions.

Babyworld.co.uk members on baby's head engaging:

▶ *Tula says:* 'If your baby is starting to engage or not it will still happen – there are no hard and fast rules about the baby engaging and when it means you will be in labour. My midwife said that baby engaging just means that his head fits – and that could mean anything.'

▶ *Mags01 says:* 'Although second and subsequent babies often don't engage until after labour has started, it's quite possible for them to engage beforehand, and this doesn't in itself mean that labour is likely to be any quicker.'

▶ *Kela says:* 'The 'fifths' measurement is confusing, as different doctors and midwives record it differently (some record how much of the head is in the pelvis, and some record how much of it can be felt above the pelvis), It's unusual to be 0/5 before labour has started, as usually the head doesn't go that far down in the pelvis until you're in labour!'

▶ *Pip180 says:* 'I think babies can pop in and out of the pelvis in second pregnancies – something to do with the muscles having been stretched previously which gives them more space to hover around the brim of the pelvis.'

▶ *LoriP says:* 'With my daughter, I went into labour and her head wasn't engaged. It actually engaged early on in labour. Incidentally I was told I was having a huge baby and that the head size was enormous and that's why it wouldn't engage. I was advised to consider a c-section. I ended up with a 6 hour labour and a 6lb 11oz baby so I'm glad I didn't.'

See also:

First signs of labour – page 180

Babyworld.co.uk link: **www.babyworld.co.uk/faq**

"I'm worried that I'll go overdue and will have to be induced. Isn't there anything else I can try to bring on labour?"

BRINGING ON LABOUR

The last few weeks of pregnancy can feel like the longest of your life. So it's no real comfort to know that there's very little you can do to change things – it really is a case of letting nature take its course. Going beyond your due date can be frustrating, and there are medical procedures that may help you avoid an induction (see box).

A lack of evidence doesn't stop some people swearing by their own 'remedies'. These range from the pleasurable (nipple stimulation, sexual intercourse) to the edible (spicy food, pineapple, raspberry leaf tea to tone the uterus (not recommended before 30-32 weeks, and not at all for women with a history of premature labour)) to the downright uncomfortable (bumpy car rides, long walks) but none of them have any real scientific research behind them. Try them if it makes you feel that you're 'doing your bit' but don't do anything dangerous or strenuous that may harm your baby. Your best bet is to try and relax; eat well, rest, exercise sensibly and enjoy the last few weeks of pregnancy. Take this chance to prepare yourself, emotionally and physically, for the birth of your baby.

Babyworld.co.uk members on bringing on labour:

▶ *Tolmie says:* 'I have tried everything with my babies and nothing worked – I ate a whole fresh pineapple, hot curries, oil in the bath, foot pressure points, raspberry leaf tea, very uncomfortable sex – I could go on. I'm not even bothering this time.'

▶ *NiaF says:* 'Two different people suggested a bumpy car ride. One girl said she had done that and then gone into labour the next day. I wouldn't drive yourself though!'

▶ *Parilo says:* 'I went for hour-long walks, did kerb walking (one foot on the road, one on the kerb) and spent the evenings doing figures of eight with my hips in the gym ball. I hated all of it, but at least I felt I was doing something.'

▶ *Kato says:* 'I have two friends who have gone into labour following a fight with their partners. Both stormed out of the house crying and went into labour half way down the street.'

▶ *Sali says:* 'With my son I was induced at 40+10. I had tried the following to get him moving: ate fresh pineapple; twiddled my nipples three times per day; sex, sex and more sex; several curries; lots of long walks; acupuncture; reflexology; two failed and one successful sweep (earlier on the day I was induced) as well as generally begging and pleading with the baby to shift his lazy backside. I also drank raspberry leaf tea regularly from about 30 weeks.'

A helping hand

A cervical sweep (also known as sweeping or stripping the membranes), which is usually done in conjunction with a cervical stretch, is a procedure carried out by a midwife or doctor when a woman is overdue, in an attempt to trigger labour. The latest research does show that there is a 17 per cent decrease in women needing to be formally induced following a stretch and sweep, but adds that this procedure can be very uncomfortable and may cause irregular contractions and sometimes a small amount of bleeding. However, formal methods of induction can be just as uncomfortable.

See also:
Sex in later pregnancy – page 124
Trying alternative remedies – page 136
Induction – page 178
Babyworld.co.uk link: **www.babyworld.co.uk/faq**

"My baby is overdue and I may have to be induced – what are the options and what should I expect?"

INDUCTION

The main reason for induction of labour is going overdue. Different hospitals have their own criteria for how long past your due dates they will wait before inducing, but it is usually between 10 and 14 days as the placental function can dramatically decline after this, putting the baby at risk. There are other reasons for induction (sometimes pre-term, but rarely before 37 weeks) including diabetes, pre-eclampsia, or if your waters break before labour starts. Concerns for the baby's health and wellbeing may also affect whether and when you may be induced.

When induction is considered, your doctor or midwife should discuss all your options before any decision is reached. They should explain the procedures involved and whether there are any risks to you or your baby. You are within your rights to decline induction but make sure you are aware of the full facts as to why it has been suggested. If you have had a previous caesarean or have had more than five babies this may affect whether induction is recommended.

There are three main medical ways to induce labour. Some women will need more than one of these to get labour going and it may take a couple of days for your baby to be born. In all cases, you will almost certainly need to remain in hospital until the birth. Prostaglandin gel or pessaries can be placed in the vagina to ripen the cervix. About 50 per cent of women who are given pessaries for induction go into labour. For some, pessaries don't work and they need to either have their waters broken and/or a Syntocinon drip to induce labour.

Induction may lead to a greater risk of caesarean if the woman is being induced because of pre-eclampsia, or if the baby is not growing well in the uterus. Induced labours can also be fast and furious. You'll need to be prepared to cope with sudden, strong contractions – it may be wise to reconsider your choices of pain relief . Sometimes a quick labour can distress the baby, leading to emergency caesarean or assisted delivery.

Babyworld.co.uk members on induction:

▶ *KariL says:* 'So many women are induced and accept the decision without doing any research. My view is that babies come when they are ready. Induction should be used for cases where there is a genuine medical reason. Too many beds are being filled up with women who have suffered complications caused by induction such as c-section or forceps deliveries.'

▶ *Tula says:* 'I really liked the fact I knew what was going on – none of that 'what's that twinge' stuff. I had midwives all around to ask stuff, I could get my beloved epidural at 4cm when most mums seem to be still at home or stuck in a waiting room.'

▶ *Hari says:* 'Unfortunately it was clinically necessary for me to be induced. I was left in a tiny cramped cubicle in the dark on my own (my husband was not allowed to stay) in labour in the middle of the night. I was scared, alone and uncomfortable. If this is the way women get treated when they are induced it doesn't surprise me at all that it usually leads to the intervention cascade (in my case gas & air, epidural, oxytocin drip, episiotomies, forceps, tearing, breastfeeding problems). Surely it would be more cost-effective to induce women in single private rooms, with their birthing partners and all those other factors that we know help women to relax, seeing as we know that anxiety leads to pain?'

See also:

Bringing on labour – page 176
Breaking waters – page 184
Assisted deliveries – page 190
Caesarean – page 194
Babyworld.co.uk link: **www.babyworld.co.uk/faq**

"As this is my first time, how will I know I am in labour? I don't want to get all excited only to find it's a false alarm."

FIRST SIGNS OF LABOUR AND FALSE ALARMS

It's often thought that there are three 'classic' signs that you're going into labour – a 'show', breaking waters and contractions. However, with the exception of contractions, where it depends on the circumstances, these signs don't necessarily mean that labour is imminent. We'll look at breaking waters separately (see page 184), but we'll consider the other signs here.

The show. This can take various forms. Generally, it's a fairly 'solid', jelly-like or stringy mucus plug that can come away in bits over several days, or in a single lump. It may be a cloudy white colour (like mucus from anywhere else in the body), or may be pinkish, reddish or brownish. You can have a show a couple of weeks or more before labour begins. On the other hand, it's possible – and actually more common – for labour to start before you have a show.

Contractions. If the contractions are stopping and starting, they may be either pre-labour (or 'latent' labour) or false labour. Pre-labour contractions are thinning the cervix and starting to open it up. They may come in bouts, with some close together and some spaced apart. False labour is irregular contractions that aren't having any effect on the cervix. Pre-labour doesn't usually go on for more than three or four days, but false labour can continue, on and off, for a couple of weeks or more. If the contractions fall into a regular pattern, getting closer together and becoming longer and stronger, then you're likely to be in labour.

Other hints that labour is imminent include back ache, a 'dropping' feeling, low abdominal pressure, period-like pains and diarrhoea – though once again, any or all of these are common in later pregnancy and shouldn't be taken as a sure sign. If you are unsure, ring your midwife and describe your symptoms, she will be able to advise you.

Babyworld.co.uk members on the first signs of labour:

▶ *Mia says:* 'With my first it was a show, followed the next day by contractions, followed the next day by going to hospital and then finally having baby on day four. With babies two, three and four the first sign was Braxton Hicks tightenings which were accompanied by a little more 'twinge' than was normal for me. Within an hour the twinges were getting more frequent and I knew they were contractions.'

▶ *Karico says:* 'I have those long slow first stage labours that gradually build up to my waters breaking at 5cms and then I deliver within an hour, so the first signs of labour could be up to three weeks before the birth, which is annoying because for three weeks everyone is on a warning and I am waiting for it all to happen.'

▶ *Sali says:* 'I didn't have a show last time – don't know what one looks like. If I had one then it was very late on when I was already in the second stage. I definitely didn't have anything before my waters broke in the hospital. It's totally true that not everyone has a show, and true that you can have one in one pregnancy and not in another.'

▶ *Pooly9 says:* 'I'm getting contractions 4-5 minutes apart, then I'm told to go into hospital. Then NOTHING. They have gone back to being every ten minutes or so, to every couple of hours and everything in between. It's mental torture. It's so hard not to get hopeful, and finding things to occupy myself is impossible.'

See also:

Measuring contractions – page 182
Breaking waters – page 184
Babyworld.co.uk link: **www.babyworld.co.uk/faq**

"I think my contractions have started – how close together should they be before I contact the hospital or midwife?"

MEASURING CONTRACTIONS

You can get tied up in knots measuring or timing contractions as their frequency doesn't necessarily provide an indication of the progress of labour. It's hard for a first-time mum to know whether the contractions she's feeling are strong, so don't be afraid to call the maternity unit or your midwife and discuss your symptoms. They will be able to tell you what to expect and advise on the best course of action, or call you in for an examination to check how far your cervix is dilated.

Remember that contractions may begin days before labour starts in earnest, so as a general rule, if you are comfortably coping with the pain of your contractions, you might be happier at home.

Babyworld.co.uk members on measuring contractions:

▶ *Kendi says:* 'I called the midwife quite early with my third baby because my contractions were only a few minutes apart, but I was still only 3cm dilated. I never had much of a gap between them, they came at small intervals from the start and within a few hours there were no intervals at all. When labour kicked in with my first and second babies, the contractions were very close together. I have never experienced 5-10 minute gaps between contractions.'

▶ *OlliT says:* 'I didn't really bother timing them until they got quite painful and seemed to be coming very close together. When that happened I got my husband to time the gap between them and also to time how long the contractions were.'

▶ *89PDQ says:* 'With my first I was obsessed with timing contractions but I had such a slow labour over a couple of days that we just ended up going to the hospital when I felt tired and uncomfortable. With my second and third babies, I timed contractions again but found that even at three to five minutes apart, if I could breathe through them and wasn't screaming it was too early to go to hospital, so I waited until the pain became overwhelming – it was better than milling around for hours in hospital or being sent home.'

▶ *Hari says:* 'By the time I know I am in labour it's too late to measure, I just have what seems to be one-long-never-ending-rollercoaster contraction that lasts about 60 minutes. Measuring them is a good way of focusing your mind though, and it can help to know that if you are unsure whether this is it, that when they get longer, stronger and closer together then it probably is.'

▶ *Melrose says:* 'During the early stages of labour, I was having irregular contractions so I wasn't sure if it was really starting or not. I just got on with some essential chores just in case and then went to a baby shower for a friend where I silently breathed my way through a few contractions because I didn't want to get people excited.'

See also:
First signs of labour – page 180
Babyworld.co.uk link: **www.babyworld.co.uk/faq**

"I've always assumed that labour starts by your waters breaking? Is that true, and if not, when do they actually break?"

BREAKING WATERS

Up to one fifth of women at the end of pregnancy start labour by their waters breaking. There's a number of theories about why this happens, including downward pressure from the baby. Some women worry about the 'embarrassment factor' of waters breaking in public, but as the above statistic shows, the chance of breaking waters being the first sign of your labour are small. Many women find they are already in hospital by the time their waters go.

When your waters break, contractions may start straight away, but they might not. Either way, if you are at home, you should call the maternity unit to let them know. Almost 70 per cent of the women whose waters break at the start of labour will give birth within 24 hours, and almost 90 per cent will give birth within 48 hours. If they don't, there is a gradually increasing risk of infection for both mother and baby as the uterus is exposed to infection. Induction is normally the next step.

Artificial rupture of the waters is also used as a common method of induction. If the cervix is slightly open because you have had some contractions (even if you haven't felt them), it is possible to use a long hook to nick the bag of waters where they bulge down in front of your baby's head. While your waters are broken, your condition should be monitored for signs of developing an infection.

Babyworld.co.uk members on waters breaking:

▶ *Mia says:* 'When your waters break, it's possible for the fluid either to gush out – in which case, it's normally fairly clear what's happened – or to trickle out, depending on whether they break at the front of or behind the baby's head. Amniotic fluid is clear or pale straw coloured, and has a slightly sweet smell.'

▶ *Pip180 says:* 'In my first two labours, the waters didn't break until the second stage of labour. First time, the head had already crowned and the midwife was about to rupture the membrane herself when it finally went.'

▶ *Suki says:* 'Don't worry if your waters break in the supermarket – at least you won't have to clear it up! I didn't buy a mattress cover and have been lucky twice as my waters have broken in hospital.'

▶ *LaraP says:* 'We put several towels under the bed sheet. Of course my waters didn't break until I was 7cm dilated and in hospital, so it was a wasted effort! My husband also made me sit on a towel in the car – apparently waters are not good for car seats either.'

▶ *Abi46 says:* 'My waters went last time when I got up out of bed. I sat up in a very undignified, whale-like, end of term pregnant woman manner, and POP! I guess there must have been a lot of pressure from baby being forced downwards with my movement. I'm trying to use gravity this time by spending loads of time walking around, but it doesn't seem to be working.'

See also:
Induction – page 178
First signs of labour – page 180
Babyworld.co.uk link: **www.babyworld.co.uk/faq**

"I'd like to have minimal pain relief – is this possible, and if so what can I do to handle the pain of labour in other ways?"

HANDLING THE PAIN

It's understandable to be frightened of the pain of labour. But this fear can make you feel more tense and makes the pain much more acute. Learning to relax during labour will help reduce any tension and will be good for you and your baby. You can find out more at antenatal classes. Some of the key techniques are listed below:

Positions When labour starts, keep active if possible. Move around and try different positions, like leaning on the back of a chair, table or bed, kneeling down and leaning on a chair or your supporter's knees, leaning on a beanbag or a birthing ball, sitting on the toilet, going onto all fours or curling up on your left-hand side.

Breathing Most relaxation techniques focus on controlling your breathing and the key is to ensure that you breathe out properly. Try to keep your breathing even during contractions. Breathe in through your nose and out through your mouth. As you breathe out, let your shoulders sink and try to release all the tension from your body.

Massage Most women feel their contractions in the lower part of their back. Ask your birth partner to use the heel of his hand to press firmly on the bottom of your spine, massaging in small circles or to use his thumbs to massage on either side of your spine. A slow and firm massage of your shoulders can keep your breathing relaxed, and long stroking massage down your spine can help you relax.

Water Relaxing in a birthing pool, taking a long, luxurious bath, or even standing under a shower can all help to ease pain and relax your tense, aching body.

Babyworld.co.uk members on handling the pain:

▶ *Kari9 says:* 'In my opinion the best way to get through labour is mental attitude. As each contraction passes that is one less to face before you get your baby. You don't get a certificate saying how well you coped with the pain so if you want maximum pain relief get it.'

▶ *Melrose says:* 'When in the established stage of labour (or any contractions that were particularly strong) I found that the only way to get through them without tensing up, was to breathe deeply and slowly through the mouth, making an O shape (like you would blowing bubbles) and when the contraction is winding up breathe in, and while the contraction is actually hitting you breathe out.'

▶ *MaggieR says:* 'My tip on how to handle the pain is to be as relaxed as possible in familiar surroundings with as little noise as possible and as few people as possible. Even at the busiest time there were only four of us in the house, with a bit of music from the TV and I was on all fours over the ball. I can honestly say, although sore, it was relaxing and easy to handle.'

▶ *Gio says:* 'I found out I was only really unable to cope right at the height of the contraction. I found counting to ten really helped to get over the worst. Singing along to music really helped too. When I realised it was only about 10-15 seconds that I had to work hard at then I found labour a lot easier.'

See also:
Antenatal classes – page 156
Fear of labour – page 160
Considering pain relief options – page 162
Labour – page 180/188
Babyworld.co.uk link: **www.babyworld.co.uk/faq**

"What can I expect to happen once active labour begins?"

FIRST AND SECOND STAGES OF LABOUR

Without wishing to abandon you in your time of need, it's almost impossible to predict your experience of labour. Any advice given in advance is likely to be based on other people's experiences and those will be coloured by the positive and negative aspects of their own labour.

We usually talk about three stages of labour. The third stage is delivery of the placenta, which is discussed elsewhere (see page 200), but the first two stages are relatively clearly defined. Once your cervix is 3cm dilated, you are considered to be in 'active labour'. Contractions will probably be strong and fairly painful by this stage, and you may be starting to need some form of pain relief.

By the time your cervix is fully dilated (10 cm), labour can progress on to the second stage. By this time, the urge to push down may be overwhelming, and this urge can consume you. Some women talk of ascending to a different plane at this stage. Many experts argue that in a completely natural labour – where there have been no interventions – there is no dividing line between the first and second stages of labour.

The duration of active labour is thought to be an average of 12 hours for first time mums and six hours for second time mums, however, not many mums are average and labour can be significantly longer or shorter than this.

Babyworld.co.uk members on labour:

▶ *Peri says:* 'At the start, labour felt like a mild cramp in my bladder, and I tried to remember how it felt so I could tell people. The cramp came at regular intervals and gradually increased in intensity until it became like my whole lower muscle structure was working to push something out and it ached down below, then the ache became a sting as the baby started to come out and that was the worst bit. I pushed with all I had, like I was doing a huge 'number two' and once the head was out, I was there. Towards the end I got so tired, but I was 'in the zone', like no one else was there, I was so focused on myself and my mission, nothing else mattered.'

▶ *Marthasmumsays:* 'No two births will ever be the same and for every horror story you hear there will be a wonderful story. Don't get your heart too set on anything as you will be disappointed if all doesn't go to plan. I planned a natural birth with as little pain relief as possible but ended up with an emergency c-section, under general anaesthetic and was really upset by the whole thing. But as long as the end result is a baby, who are we to complain.'

▶ *KariLP says:* 'The best part for me was when the pushing came. Something primal took over and I finally felt like I was on the home stretch. I think there is something primal and instinctive about giving birth and it's a good thing to be in an environment, position and relaxed enough state to let that take over and take control of your body.'

See also:
Fear of labour – page 160
Handing the pain – page 186
Delivering the placenta – page 200
Babyworld.co.uk link: **www.babyworld.co.uk/faq**

> **"Why might I need to have a forceps or vacuum extractor delivery? How do they compare and what are the risks?"**

ASSISTED DELIVERIES

There are many reasons why an assisted delivery may be necessary. You may be too tired to be able to give birth on your own, or your uterus may be exhausted and contractions are no longer very efficient after a long labour. Your baby may have become distressed during the pushing part of labour, or isn't in the best position to be born easily (e.g. breech position). If you've had an epidural you may be finding it difficult to know when and how to push with the contractions, making the second stage of labour less efficient.

Forceps look like stainless steel salad servers. They are large and the curved ends are called blades. The forceps come in two sections and the doctor gently places the first blade round the side of your baby's head, and then the second blade round the other side. You are asked to push with your next contraction and the doctor pulls. Ventouse is a suction cap made of silicone plastic. It fits onto the baby's head like a skull cap. Once the cap has been positioned, air is sucked out of it using a vacuum device.

With forceps the mother will require effective pain relief before the delivery is carried out, she will also have to have an episiotomy. There is an additional risk of damage to the mother's bladder and bowel function and the baby may also be bruised or may suffer minor nerve damage. With a ventouse, pain relief may not be necessary. It may be possible to apply the cup to the baby's head without cutting the perineum and there is less risk of damage to the mother's vagina and bladder.

Babyworld.co.uk members on assisted deliveries:

▶ *Sasha56 says:* 'I had a ventouse delivery with my first. She was showing signs of distress and I'd done well with my long labour and really didn't want a c-section if I could help it. They put my legs up on stirrups and managed to drag her out in two pushes with a ventouse. Since I was numb I can't comment on the pain and although I did need stitches it was only a couple so I guess I was lucky. Her head was a funny shape for a few days and she was a very lazy feeder and preferred to sleep or cry those early days – someone said that was probably because she had a cracking headache!'

▶ *Tula says:* 'My last delivery was a vacuum extraction. I didn't have time to consider it and wasn't briefed or asked for an opinion, and I didn't need to be either. Sometimes you just have to trust the medical professionals to get on with it, my baby wasn't breathing and his heart had stopped – it was no time to discuss our options.'

▶ *KatiP says:* 'My second child was yanked into the world by ventouse. It wasn't needed and to this day I still feel angry. I have found that by avoiding a standard labour ward delivery and epidurals that I have also avoided the need for an assisted delivery.'

See also:
Considering pain relief options – page 166
Breech birth – page 196
Foetal distress – page 198
Babyworld.co.uk link: **www.babyworld.co.uk/faq**

"What is an episiotomy and why might I need to have one of these in labour?"

EPISIOTOMY

An episiotomy is an emergency procedure which can be used if the baby needs to be born quickly. It involves a cut in the perineum (the area between the vagina and the anus) made with scissors.

Episiotomies were once routine, and a woman having her first baby in hospital was unlikely to escape having the procedure performed. Nowadays, you will only have an episiotomy if the baby is in distress, if it is needed for an assisted delivery (with forceps or ventouse), or you are likely to tear very badly. The latter is a debatable reason, because episiotomies don't actually appear to prevent bad tears, and it is possible to tear as well as having a cut.

Most midwives have the skills to support women to avoid not only an episiotomy but also unnecessary tearing.

Research suggests that massaging your perineum with oil before birth can reduce your risk of tearing. Doing pelvic floor exercises before birth can also reduce the chances of tearing, and can help the perineum heal after the birth if any damage has occurred.

Babyworld.co.uk members on Episiotomy:

▶ *MelK says:* 'I had a small episiotomy with my third baby, and it didn't require any stitches. It was to help ease out the baby's head without tearing (he was fairly large at 9lb 10 oz). I had no problems with it at all. I'd torn with the first two babies, and had a third degree tear with my first (stitched in theatre) and minor tear with my second (required a few stitches). The episiotomy seemed to be a better option for me!'

▶ *TeriP says:* 'The midwives at the hospital all told me that it would take about 7-10 days for the cut to get better. What they meant was that it should be pain free after 7 – 10 days. The stitches take approximately 6 weeks to dissolve depending on how fast your body heals. If it is still really painful after about five days, go to the doctor and have it checked in case you have an infection.'

▶ *Marthasmum says:* 'I had on my birth plan that I preferred to tear naturally which is what I did with my first delivery using a ventouse. Fortunately it was not a big tear and only needed a couple of stitches. I do know women who have torn badly though and wish they'd opted for a neat episiotomy since stitching a bad tear is tricky and the scar tissue has remained lumpy and required further treatment since.'

See also:

Pelvic floor exercises – page 66

Assisted deliveries – page 190

Babyworld.co.uk link: **www.babyworld.co.uk/faq**

"Under what circumstances might I need a caesarean, and what are the risks and benefits?"

CAESAREAN (ELECTIVE AND EMERGENCY)

There are two kinds of caesarean. An elective caesarean is carried out before labour begins. An emergency caesarean is carried out as a result of some complication arising during labour.

You may be advised to have an elective caesarean if pre-eclampsia is threatening your health and your baby, or if you have a serious medical condition which means that you should avoid labour. Other reasons for an elective caesarean include: if you are expecting triplets or more; if the placenta is lying across the neck of your uterus; if your baby is lying across your tummy; if your baby is too big to get through your pelvis; if your baby is in the breech position (see page 196 for more information on breech babies and caesareans).

An emergency caesarean might be necessary after labour has started because your baby is not coping well with contractions or if the cervix stops dilating so that both mother and baby become exhausted. If the placenta starts to come away from the wall of the uterus or if the baby does not move down into the pelvis, an emergency caesarean may also be advised.

Most hospitals prefer to give regional anaesthetics (spinal block or epidural) though a general anaesthetic may be used for an emergency caesarean. Post-operative recovery is slower than recovery from a natural birth, you may require painkillers and will be unable to lift heavy objects or drive for at least six weeks after the surgery. Some women also experience negative feelings after a caesarean, including a sense of personal failure. With time, it should be easier to appreciate that this is a harsh self-judgement – carrying a baby for nine months is enough of an achievement for anyone, and the manner of delivery is nowhere near as important as the safe arrival of the baby.

Babyworld.co.uk members on caesareans:

▶ *KT90 says:* 'I am against non-medically necessary caesareans and most could be avoided if women were supported in labour so epidurals were not needed, routine inductions for dubious reasons avoided, and if women were just given the confidence in their bodies to give birth. I think this confidence is often undermined by the medical profession.'

▶ *Mia says:* 'Things don't always go to plan and I think that needs to be remembered. Don't put pressure on yourself to have a perfect labour, if things don't work out it doesn't mean that you haven't succeeded. Even though I had an emergency caesarean and couldn't give birth to my son naturally I was still the proudest mummy in the world. With my second son I had an elective and it was still a very relaxing, beautiful experience.'

▶ *Tolmie says:* 'Caesareans should not be necessary for second or subsequent birth, and VBAC (Vaginal Birth After Caesarean) is usually far safer (even after two or three) – but women are not usually given the correct statistics to make this decision and doctors often prefer to encourage a repeat caesarean.'

▶ *HelenJ says:* 'Women need to be told the risks of caesareans and they are not being told. I had two ectopic pregnancies caused by scar tissue from my caesareans and these were a shock to me as I had no idea that caesareans could cause this. It's quite a common occurrence though – and due to the rise in caesareans, ectopics caused by this are increasing too.'

See also:
Pre-eclampsia – page 106
Breech birth – page 196
Babyworld.co.uk link: **www.babyworld.co.uk/faq**

"My baby is in the breech position – will it definitely stay this way, or is there anything I can do to shift it?"

BREECH BIRTH

Breech babies are the most common problem when it comes to foetal positioning. Around 15 per cent of babies are breech at 32 weeks, but only two to three per cent are breech at birth. From 36 weeks, the chances of the baby turning decreases significantly. At this stage, you will be referred to a consultant to discuss your options. A scan will check the baby's exact position and weight, and see if you have a low-lying placenta, which can sometimes cause a breech position.

It is possible to manoeuvre a baby from breech position to head-first. This procedure is called external cephalic version (ECV) and is usually done after 37 weeks, with a 50 per cent success rate. The doctor will place their hands on your uterus and guide your baby through a forward somersault. Some doctors use a drug to help your uterus relax, especially for first-time mums. The procedure may feel uncomfortable but shouldn't be painful. An ECV is relatively safe, but the baby's heartbeat will be checked before and after to check everything is OK.

There is an increasing tendency for babies who remain in the breech position to be delivered by caesarean rather than vaginally. This is due to the risk of problems such as fractures, asphyxia, and brain haemorrhage with vaginal breech birth. Not all hospitals have a strict policy on this and each case should be viewed individually. Many doctors and midwives believe vaginal births are possible for some breech babies, although intervention, in the form of forceps delivery, is quite common.

Babyworld.co.uk members on moving a breech baby:

▶ *Lilkat says:* 'To encourage your baby to turn head down, you could try the 'bum-in-the-air' techniques. These involve kneeling with your forearms on the floor, your head down, and your bottom up, or lying on your back with your feet on the floor, your knees bent up and three or four pillows under your bottom. Do it for 10-15 minutes two or three times a day. The theory is they tip the baby away from your pelvis, so that when you're upright again, the baby's head will drop down by force of gravity.'

▶ *Lua says:* 'Alternative therapies – acupuncture, reflexology and homeopathy – all claim some success at turning breech babies, but you'd need to speak to a qualified practitioner about these.'

Babyworld.co.uk members on breech birth:

▶ *Maxie says:* 'I think some midwives have lost the art of breech delivery. If this could be regained then breech delivery could happen more often. As it is women who want a breech birth tend to opt for an independent midwife – since these midwives retain the skill of breech delivery.'

Kaylo9's story

'I have delivered a breech presentation vaginally. My consultant refused to deliver me so I changed to one that would consider it. We tried to turn the baby manually but he wouldn't have it. After some discussion and scans of different sorts it was decided that the baby was a complete breech and that I had large enough internal parameters to attempt delivery.

When I went into labour I rang and informed them that I was coming in and to be appointed a midwife with experience of delivering breech babies. I was adamant that I would attempt this without a doctor. During early labour I discussed that I didn't want any pain relief and needed to be upright. The whole thing was no more painful than a standard labour.'

See also:

Caesarean – page 194

Babyworld.co.uk link: **www.babyworld.co.uk/faq**

"What causes foetal distress in labour, and how can it be prevented?"

FOETAL DISTRESS

Midwife says: Foetal distress is an unfortunate and worrying part of labour for a small minority of parents. Broadly speaking, what foetal distress means is that the baby is not receiving enough oxygen for some reason. These reasons include the cord being compressed or entangled, a problem with the placenta, the mother being flat on her back and this restricting the blood flow to the baby, and the effects of medical procedures, such as the use of drugs to induce or speed up labour.

The most common sign of foetal distress is the baby's heart rate dropping, so in order to keep a check on this, your midwife will ask listen to your baby's heart at frequent intervals during labour, using a handheld listening device, although in certain circumstances, it is necessary for the baby's heart rate to be monitored continuously with electronic equipment. If the monitoring reveals that the baby is showing signs of distress, steps are taken to help increase the flow of oxygen to the baby, but if these are not effective, it becomes necessary for the baby to be born as quickly as possible, either instrumentally (using forceps or ventouse) or by caesarean.

In many cases, the cause of foetal distress isn't something that can be prevented, but you can help to keep a good supply of oxygen going to your baby during labour by not lying on your back and relaxing as much as possible.

Babyworld.co.uk members on foetal distress:

▶ *Luma says:* 'I had an epidural with my daughter and there were a couple of times where her heart rate decelerated so the midwife told me that they couldn't increase the dosage of the epidural as it was causing the baby some distress. When her head was delivered, the cord was around her neck. I didn't know this and the staff never mentioned it, not even after delivery. When she was born, she wasn't actually in any distress at all as her APGAR scores were fine. However, this is one situation where I believe it's best to err on the side of caution especially as my husband tells me that the cord was quite tight around my daughter's neck.'

▶ *Tez says:* 'My baby's heart rate caused the midwives some concern so they broke my waters which were discoloured with meconium, another sign that she was in distress. Things were speeded up further and I then experienced 3 hours of sheer agony from contractions, constant monitoring but finally a healthy baby born naturally. I wouldn't recommend induction and interference to anyone but sometimes it's necessary... take my advice though – don't be brave and stick the pain – just ask for an epidural, I wish I had!'

▶ *Suki8 says:* 'I believe that foetal distress can be avoided in some cases by steering clear of interventions and therefore not starting a cascade of interventions. Staying at home, understanding what is happening and using more natural methods of pain relief can help to avoid further interventions. Although I do understand that there are times when there is no avoiding it, it's not all our fault!'

See also:
Managing complications in labour – page 202
Babyworld.co.uk link: **www.babyworld.co.uk/faq**

> **"What are the pros and cons of having a managed delivery of the placenta?"**

DELIVERING THE PLACENTA

The delivery of the placenta – known as the third stage of labour – can seem like an anticlimax, as the baby is already born. But there are important decisions to be made regarding this part of the process and if you have specific opinions on how you want your entire labour to be managed, you should give this serious thought beforehand.

There are two ways in which the placenta can be delivered. One is a natural delivery when the placenta is left to come out without any assistance from your midwife. This usually takes around 15-20 minutes, but may take up to an hour. The other is known as a 'managed' third stage. This involves having an injection of a substance called syntometrine (or, in some hospitals, syntocinon) once your baby's head and first shoulder have been born to control the delivery of the placenta, with the midwife helping to get it out. The placenta comes out in about 5-10 minutes. A managed delivery reduces the amount of bleeding that occurs when the placenta detaches from the wall of the uterus.

Some hospitals offer a managed third stage as a matter of routine, other hospitals will ask you beforehand how you'd like to deliver the placenta. If you don't want the injection, say so on your birth plan so that the midwife knows in advance. An injection is strongly advised in the following circumstances: If you've been anaemic in pregnancy; if you've had any bleeding in pregnancy; if you've had a drip to start or speed up labour; if you've had pain-killing drugs or an epidural; if you've had forceps or ventouse; if you have more than one baby; if you've had a very long labour; and if you have raised blood pressure.

Babyworld.co.uk members on delivering the placenta:

▶ *Sali says:* 'I had the injection with my first baby – beforehand, I was all for the natural route, but having spent over two hours pushing her out, I just wanted a cup of tea and toast! This time, I'm in two minds – my midwife says that with a natural placenta expulsion, you bleed more initially but less in the following days, and vice versa with the injection.'

▶ *MiaG says:* 'Delivering the placenta naturally isn't more painful. In fact, because with the injection, the midwife has to pull on the cord in order to help the placenta out, that can actually be more uncomfortable.'

▶ *Pip180 says:* 'If you've had an intervention and drug-free delivery then you might want to finish things off naturally. Particularly if you can put the baby straight to the breast, as the nipple stimulation encourages the uterus to contract and expel the placenta.'

▶ *Gio says:* 'I've put in my birth plan that I would like the placenta delivered naturally and the cord cut only after it's stopped pulsing. I don't see why I can't let nature do its stuff if everything is going well. We were also told at the antenatal classes, that the main disadvantage of having the injection is that the midwife then only has 15 minutes to get the placenta out before the cervix starts closing, so she can get quite stressed out about it.'

▶ *Suki says:* 'I turned down the syntometrine for my first labour and then haemorrhaged. I was told that this was because the uterus was large (the baby weighed 10lbs). I needed a drip for several hours until the bleeding settled. For my next two babies I had home births, so I had the syntometrine to be sure I wouldn't haemorrhage again as I'd probably have had to go into hospital afterwards.'

See also:

Babyworld.co.uk link: **www.babyworld.co.uk/faq**

"Will the medical team always respect my wishes, or could there come a stage when they just take over and do what they think is best?"

MANAGING COMPLICATIONS IN LABOUR

Not all labours are straightforward, and those that go on for many hours or face specific complications may result in a course of action different to that defined in your birth plan.

Where possible all decisions during labour should be discussed and agreed with you. But if agreement cannot be reached and the medical team is insistent on a course of action, it may be necessary to defer to their expertise. If you're uncomfortable with this ask yourself the following questions – have they explained any procedures and their likely outcomes fully? Have they consulted your birth plan and your birth partner to see whether any alternatives could be used? If the answers are yes, then you are unlikely to be in a position to refuse their recommendations.

Briefing your birth partner, writing a detailed birth plan and talking through your concerns with the attending medical team at an early stage will all help to reassure you that you're in the best hands. But given the unpredictable nature of labour, it is essential to go into the experience with an open mind and a flexible approach.

Babyworld.co.uk members on managing complications in labour:

▶ *Bex says:* 'During my second labour, the induction failed and I was in the unfortunate situation of arguing with a doctor. I didn't want a caesarean, and was being bullied into opting for one. I found it hard to get my opinion across without being forceful, as I felt the doctor was trying to manipulate me constantly into doing what she felt was the easiest thing.'

▶ *Sali says:* 'It can be very difficult to communicate with the medical staff. In my experience, they don't always believe that you are a rational thinking human being capable of making your own decisions. This is where it's important for your birth partner to know what it is that you want and to be able to argue on your behalf.'

▶ *Megs says:* 'You are too busy with the business of labour to be able to effectively communicate your desires and requests. When I was in the second stage of labour, if they had told me that they needed to remove my leg at the knee in order to get my baby out, I would have agreed. I'd have regretted it later but at the time all you want to do is get that baby out.'

▶ *Kia70 says:* 'I am a firm believer in the 'you get more flies with honey' approach to communication and I have found that if you treat the medical staff with respect (as you would like to be treated) you are more likely to get assistance and agreement than if you are confrontational. Of course, there are always exceptions!'

▶ *Fideli says:* 'When I had complications in labour I trusted them to do what was necessary for a healthy outcome. If you feel uncomfortable with your attending medic then you need to say so and change before you have to rely on them to 'know' what you would want to do. I feel that often women can 'feel' what another woman would want, or need. That's why a good midwife is crucial.'

See also:
Writing a birth plan – page 168
Choosing and briefing a birth partner – page 170
Foetal distress – page 198
Babyworld.co.uk link: **www.babyworld.co.uk/faq**

"I've been warned that I might bleed after the birth. How much loss should I expect and for how long?"

BLEEDING AFTER THE BIRTH

Blood loss following the birth varies from woman to woman. Some stop bleeding within a week or so, while others continue to bleed off and on for six weeks. It is unusual to still be losing lochia – the name for this mixture of blood and mucus – after six weeks, but not unknown.

Lochia are generally heavy and red for the first few days, becoming lighter and more brownish as the days pass. Some women find blood loss gets heavier and turns bright red again for a day or so in the second week when they become more active. Lochia have a characteristic 'sweet' smell, which should not be offensive or strong. If other people notice the smell, there may be a problem. Your GP can examine your cervix for the presence of an ectropion – a patch of moist, delicate cells on the outside of the cervix. This is extremely common, and not generally a problem unless the area becomes infected or bleeds following intercourse.

You are likely to bleed more with each subsequent child, and the risk increases significantly after baby number three. The muscles of your uterus become more lax each time you are pregnant and so your body's natural defence against haemorrhage is compromised. It is your uterus's ability to contract strongly after the placenta comes away that stops you bleeding.

Babyworld.co.uk members on bleeding after the birth:

▶ *Kat5 says:* 'You will definitely need maternity pads, I had to use two together for the first day. Trust me, you will bleed like never before! I was actually quite frightened when I had a shower after the birth, my mum called the midwife as there was so much blood in the shower, but she said it was perfectly normal straight after the birth.'

▶ *Tolmie says:* 'Nobody told me about the amount of bleeding (of the period-like variety) you have after a natural birth. I got a bit of a shock when mine lasted 10 weeks after birth but was told this can be quite normal. Mine was also very heavy. I know it won't be the same in everyone's case but forewarned is forearmed!'

▶ *Marthasmum says:* 'As breastfeeding helps the uterus to contract to its pre-pregnancy size quicker you do tend to bleed more heavily if breastfeeding. It was so bad sometimes that every time I stood up I needed to change. I also bled for 6 weeks which is quite a long time.'

▶ *TeriK says:* 'A lot of women these days are not used to pads anymore. The maternity ones do seem better if you have stitches as they don't have as much plastic in them as night-time pads which can affect your stitches. You can bleed up to 6 weeks although most women seem to tail off after two. If you don't want to use maternity pads get the most absorbent ones you can. Or you could get a mixture of maternity and normal and see which you find best.'

See also:
Packing for the hospital – page 172
Babyworld.co.uk link: **www.babyworld.co.uk/faq**

CONTACT US

You're welcome to contact White Ladder Press if you have any questions or comments for either us or the authors. Please use whichever of the following routes suits you.

Phone: 01803 813343

Email: enquiries@whiteladderpress.com

Fax: 01803 813928

Address: White Ladder Press, Great Ambrook, Near Ipplepen, Devon TQ12 5UL

Website: www.whiteladderpress.com

WHAT CAN OUR WEBSITE DO FOR YOU?

If you want more information about any of our books, you'll find it at **www.whiteladderpress.com**. In particular you'll find extracts from each of our books, and reviews of those that are already published. We also run special offers on future titles if you order online before publication. And you can request a copy of our free catalogue.

Many of our books have links pages, useful addresses and so on relevant to the subject of the book. You'll also find out a bit more about us and, if you're a writer yourself, you'll find our submission guidelines for authors. So please check us out and let us know if you have any comments, questions or suggestions.

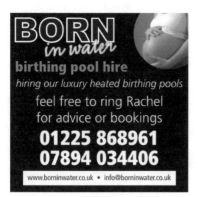
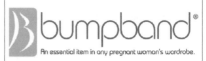

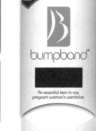
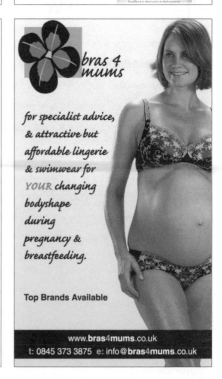

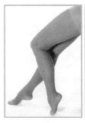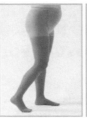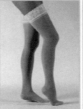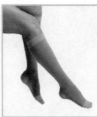
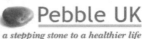
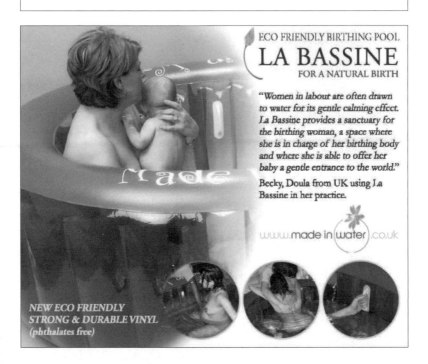

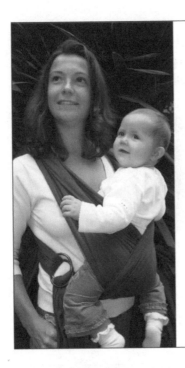
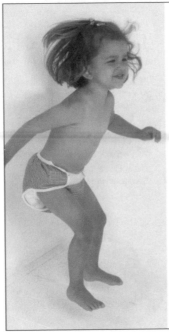

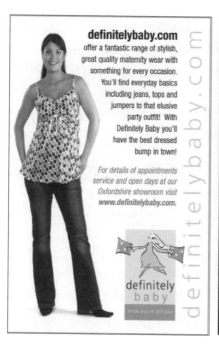
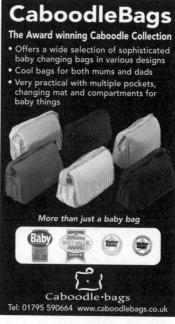

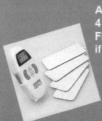
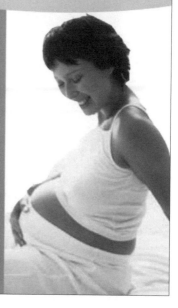

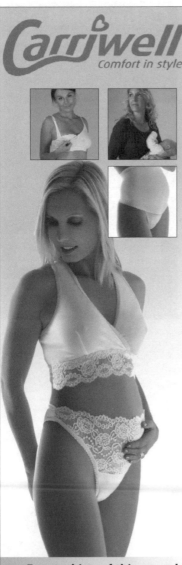
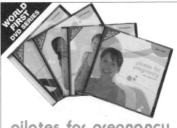
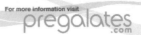
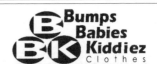

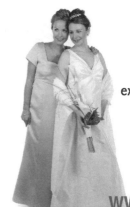

From **Lad** to **Dad**

How to survive as a pregnant father

"Stephen Giles describes the fears and frustrations of impending fatherhood with honesty and humour, along with practical help and advice." **Lawrence Dallaglio**

You've done it – she's pregnant. Now all you have to do is sit back, put your feet up and wait for the congratulations of friends and family. Right?

Wrong. Suddenly it's all about her and you're relegated to the sidelines, facing nine long months of getting lost in her ever expanding shadow.

So forget the laid back lifestyle (you'll be too busy waiting on her every whim). Forget late night socialising (she'll be too tired). And forget sex, obviously. At least in any form you'd recognise. Instead you've got to learn a whole new role, and fast.

Now at least you have one fellow traveller to take your side and give you the attention you deserve. Stephen Giles has charted his own journey from lad to dad and shares his ignorance, humiliations, frustrations, inadequacies and downright sodding terror. Along the way he guides you through the minefield of dismissive midwives, scary hospital visits, mood swings (hers as well as yours), and the looming prospect of having to reinvent yourself as a halfway decent dad.

He also passes on the answers to many of his own questions, along with a mass of practical and realistic advice, and reassures you that if he can survive as a pregnant father, so can you. In fact not only can you survive, but you can emerge at the end of it all feeling bloody fantastic.

"Here is the proof that you are not alone. Nor are you useless, powerless or redundant. You're the daddy, almost. And absolutely nothing beats that."

£7.99

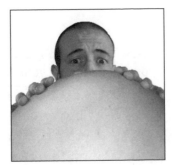

Babies

for Beginners

Roni Jay

"A perfect first book for all new mums and dads confused by parenthood." *Pregnancy*

At last, here is the book for every new parent who's never been quite sure what a cradle cap is and whether you need one. *Babies for Beginners* cuts away the crap – the unnecessary equipment, the overfussy advice – and gives you the absolute basics of babycare: keep the baby alive, at all costs, and try to stop it getting too hungry.

From bedtime to bathtime, mealtime to playtime, this book highlights the core *objective* of each exercise (for example, get the baby bathed) and the *key focus* (don't drown it). By exploding the myths around each aspect of babycare, the book explains what is necessary and what is a bonus; what equipment is essential and what you can do without.

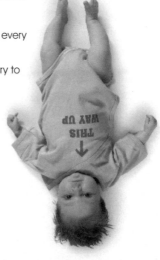

Babies for Beginners is the perfect book for every first time mother who's confused by all the advice and can't believe it's really necessary to spend that much money. And it's the ultimate guide for every father looking for an excuse to get out of ante-natal classes.

Roni Jay is a professional author whose books include *KIDS & Co: winning business tactics for every family*. She is the mother of three young children, and stepmother to three grown up ones.

This edition contains new material

£7.99

You're the **Daddy**

From nappy mess to happiness in one year
The art of being a great dad

Stephen **Giles**

And you thought pregnancy was a steep learning curve? Once the baby is born, your life turns upside down. Sure, a lot of the changes are great, but they're all new and you set out with barely a clue how to cope. Life is packed with new challenges to face and new skills to learn.

That's why you need a friend and guide to reassure you and hold your hand through that crucial first year.

A follow-up to his popular and highly entertaining *From Lad to Dad How to survive as a pregnant father*, Stephen Giles now sets out his progress through the first year of his baby's life. Once again he tells his story in journal form with great humour, and plenty of practical ideas and advice for other first time fathers on topics such as:

- the conflict between work pressure and sleepless nights
- division of labour at home
- being the breadwinner, the main carer or any combination of the two
- your changing relationship with your partner
- keeping 'competitive dad syndrome' under control

Stephen will help you ensure that by the end of your first year not only will you be able to change a nappy in your sleep (should you be lucky enough to get any) but, more importantly, you'll have mastered the art of being a great dad.

£7.99

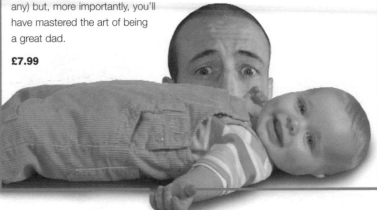

Order form

You can order any of our books via any of the contact routes on page 207, including on our website. Or fill out the order form below and fax it or post it to us.

We'll normally send your copy out by first class post within 24 hours (but please allow five days for delivery). We don't charge postage and packing within the UK. Please add £1 per book for postage outside the UK.

Title (Mr/Mrs/Miss/Ms/Dr/Lord etc)

Name

Address

Postcode

Daytime phone number

Email

No. of copies	Title	Price	Total £
	Postage and packing £1 per book (outside the UK only):		
		TOTAL:	

Please either send us a cheque made out to White Ladder Press Ltd or fill in the credit card details below.

Type of card ☐ Visa ☐ Mastercard ☐ Switch

Card number

Start date (if on card)   Expiry date   Issue no (Switch)

Security code (last 3 digits on reverse of card)

Name as shown on card

Signature

INDEX